Sheila J. Baker

DASH DIET COOKBOOK

Easy and Healthy Recipes with Specific Nutritional Values. Change Your Eating Habits to Lower Your Blood Pressure and Lose Weight with Low Sodium Recipes

SHEILA J. BAKER

© Copyright 2020 - All rights reserved.

The content contained within this book may not be reproduced, duplicated or transmitted without direct written permission from the author or the publisher. Under no circumstances will any blame or legal responsibility be held against the publisher, or author, for any damages, reparation, or monetary loss due to the information contained within this book. Either directly or indirectly.

Legal Notice:

This book is copyright protected. This book is only for personal use. You cannot amend, distribute, sell, use, quote or paraphrase any part, or the content within this book, without the consent of the author or publisher.

Disclaimer Notice:

Please note the information contained within this document is for educational and entertainment purposes only. All effort has been executed to present accurate, up to date, and reliable, complete information. No warranties of any kind are declared or implied. Readers acknowledge that the author is not engaging in the rendering of legal, financial, medical or professional advice. The content within this book has been derived from various sources. Please consult a licensed professional before attempting any techniques outlined in this book.

By reading this document, the reader agrees that under no circumstances is the author responsible for any losses, direct or indirect, which are incurred as a result of the use of information contained within this document, including, but not limited to, errors, omissions, or inaccuracies.

Table of Contents

INTRODUCTION 7

CHAPTER 1: UNDERSTANDING THE DASH DIET 9
- Origin of the DASH Diet 9
- Health Advantages of the DASH Diet 10
- The DASH Dietary Program 11
- Research-Based Benefits of DASH Dieting 12
- Ten Reasons Why the DASH Diet Truly Works 12

CHAPTER 2: BREAKFAST & SMOOTHIES 15
- Yogurt & Banana Muffins 16
- Berry Quinoa Bowls 17
- Pineapple Green Smoothie 18
- Peanut Butter & Banana Smoothie 19
- Pumpkin-Hazelnut Tea Cake 20
- Raspberry Chocolate Scones 21
- Banana Almond Smoothie 22
- Blueberry Banana Muffins 23
- Easy Buckwheat Crepes 24
- Peanut Butter Oats in the Jar 25
- Fruit Smoothie 26
- Green Smoothie 27
- Heart-Friendly Sweet Potato-Oats Waffles 28
- Rhubarb Pecan Muffins 29
- Whole-Wheat Pretzels 30
- Mushroom Frittata 31
- Cheesy Omelet 32
- Ginger Congee 33
- Egg Melts 34

CHAPTER 3: SALADS 35
- Spring Greens Salad 36
- Tuna Salad 37
- Fish Salad 38
- Salmon Salad 39
- Arugula Salad with Shallot 40
- Watercress Salad 41
- Seafood Arugula Salad 42
- Smoked Salad 43
- Avocado Salad 44
- Berry Salad with Shrimps 45
- Sliced Mushrooms Salad 46
- Tender Green Beans Salad 47
- Spinach and Chicken Salad 48
- Cilantro Salad 49
- Iceberg Salad 50
- Seafood Salad with Grapes 51

CHAPTER 4: SOUPS & STEWS 53
- Pumpkin Cream Soup 54
- Zucchini Noodles Soup 55
- Grilled Tomatoes Soup 56
- Chicken Oatmeal Soup 57
- Celery Cream Soup 58
- Cauliflower Soup 59
- Buckwheat Soup 60
- Parsley Soup 61
- Tomato Bean Soup 62
- Red Kidney Beans Soup 63
- Pork Soup 64
- Curry Soup 65
- Yellow Onion Soup 66
- Garlic Soup 67

CHAPTER 5: VEGAN & VEGETARIAN 69
- Chickpea Curry 70
- Quinoa Bowl 71
- Vegan Meatloaf 72
- Loaded Potato Skins 73
- Vegan Shepherd Pie 74
- Cauliflower Steaks 75
- Quinoa Burger 76
- Cauliflower Tots 77
- Zucchini Soufflé 78
- Honey Sweet Potato Bake 79
- Lentil Quiche 80
- Corn Patties 81
- Tofu Stir Fry 82
- Mac Stuffed Sweet Potatoes 83
- Tofu Tikka Masala 84
- Tofu Parmigiana 85
- Mushroom Stroganoff 86
- Eggplant Croquettes 87
- Stuffed Portobello 88
- Chile Rellenos 89
- Garbanzo Stir Fry 90

CHAPTER 6: FISH & SEAFOOD 91

- Halibut with Tomato, Basil, and Oregano Salsa ...92
- Roasted Salmon with Chives and Tarragon 93
- Grilled Shrimp Salad with Orange Vinaigrette 94
- Halibut with Radish Slices 95
- Green Onion Salmon 96
- Broccoli and Cod Mash....................................97
- Greek Style Salmon 98
- Spicy Ginger Seabass 99
- Yogurt Shrimps 100
- Aromatic Salmon with Fennel Seeds 101
- Shrimp Quesadillas...102
- The OG Tuna Sandwich 103
- Easy To Make Mussels 104
- Chili-Rubbed Tilapia with Asparagus & Lemon.....105
- Parmesan-Crusted Fish...................................106
- Lemon Swordfish 107
- Spiced Scallops 108
- Shrimp Puttanesca 109
- Curry Snapper 110
- Grouper with Tomato Sauce 111
- Braised Seabass 112

CHAPTER 7: PORK & BEEF................................ 113

- Beef Stroganoff..114
- Pork Roast with Orange Sauce 116
- Southwestern Steak.......................................117
- Tender Pork Medallions..................................118
- Garlic Pork Meatballs 119
- Fajita Pork Strips 120
- Pepper Pork Tenderloins.................................121
- Spiced Beef 122
- Tomato Beef 123
- Hoisin Pork 124
- Sage Beef Loin 125
- Beef Chili..126
- Celery Beef Stew 127
- Beef Skillet 128
- Hot Beef Strips..129
- Sloppy Joe 130

CHAPTER 8: SNACKS, SIDES & DESSERTS............131

- Summer Squash Ribbons with Lemon and Ricotta 132
- Sautéed Kale with Tomato and Garlic 133
- Roasted Broccoli with Tahini Yogurt Sauce 134
- Green Beans with Pine Nuts and Garlic 135
- Roasted Harissa Carrots..................................136
- Toasted Almond Ambrosia 137
- Apple Dumplings 138
- Almond Rice Pudding 139
- Apples and Cream Shake 140
- Baked Stuffed Apples.....................................141
- Apricot Biscotti 142
- Apple & Berry Cobbler.....................................143
- Mixed Fruit Compote Cups...............................144
- Oatmeal Surprise Cookies................................145
- Almond & Apricot Crisp 146
- Blueberry Apple Cobbler 147

CHAPTER 9: MEASUREMENT CONVERSIONS 149

CONCLUSION 151

Introduction

Generally speaking, most people who are looking to start the DASH diet are people who suffer from high blood pressure themselves or have a family member that does.

Men are more likely to have hypertension issues, especially after the age of 45, and a significant amount of patients with diabetes will experience these symptoms as well. Also, put at risk are individuals who are overweight. However, hypertension can happen to anyone.

DASH is an acronym for Dietary Approaches to Stop Hypertension. The diet is centered on eating a balanced combination of lean meats, vegetables, whole grains, and fruits, and keeping sodium intake between two-thirds and one tablespoon of salt per day depending on the reasons for starting the diet and the results you are seeking.

The DASH diet also focuses on keeping fats, added sugars, and red meat to a lower level. As with all diets, there is a happy medium for keeping true to the diet.

When you experience the symptoms of hypertension for extended amounts of time, you are more at risk for heart disease, kidney issues, and higher glucose levels leading to diabetes. You also are at a higher risk of early mortality.

However, following the simple to understand guidelines of the DASH Diet will help to bring your blood pressure numbers to a more manageable level and help you to be healthier in the long run, bringing your chances of living a much more fulfilling life for you.

When you work towards your goals on the DASH Diet, you will start to see the results rather quickly which will help you to keep your willpower working towards your personal goals.

CHAPTER 1:

Understanding the Dash Diet

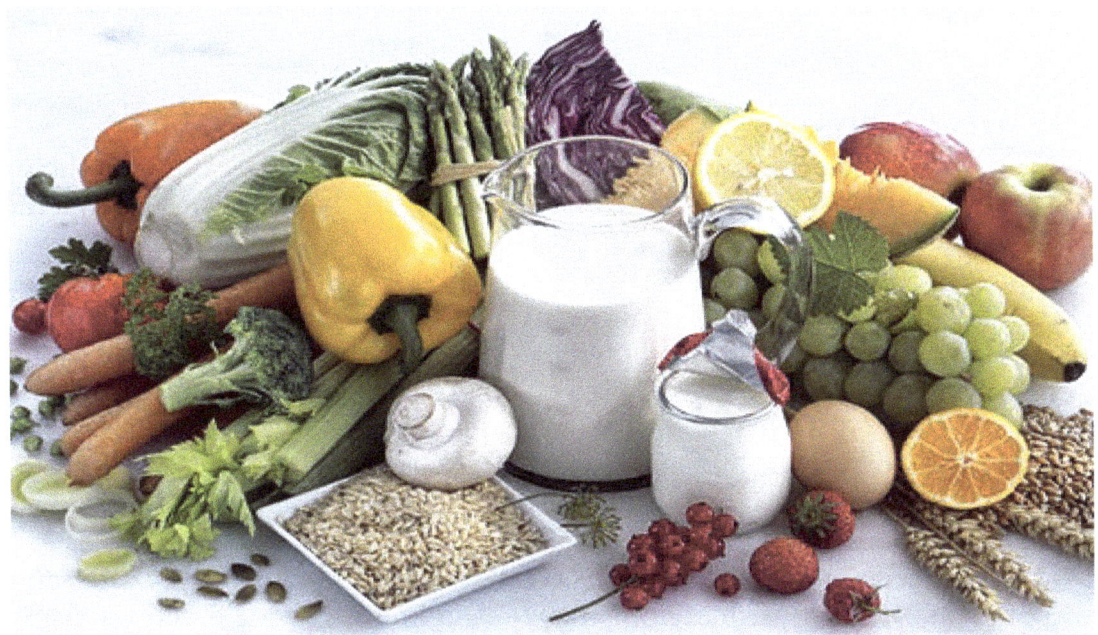

Dietary Approaches to Stop Hypertension is one of the most effective organic treatments of all health problems related to high blood pressure or fluid build-up in the body. These approaches come with a complete program, which places emphasis on the diet as well as lifestyle changes. Commonly called the DASH diet, the major target is to reduce the sodium content of your diet by omitting table salt directly or reducing the intake through other ingredients. There are two minerals that work against each other to maintain the body fluid balance: those are sodium and potassium. In perfect proportions, these two control the release and retention of fluids in the body. In the case of environmental or genetic complexities or a high sodium diet, the balance is disturbed so much that it puts our heart at risk by elevating systolic and diastolic blood pressures.

Origin of the DASH Diet

This dietary plan came to the knowledge of nutritionists after several research studies were conducted to treat hypertension focused on diet in order to avoid medication's side effects. It was seen as a way to reduce the blood pressure using healthy, nourishing food and following an active routine. The main goal was to cure hypertension, so it was soon termed as the Dietary Approaches to Stop Hypertension (DASH). However, its broad-scale effects showed greater efficiency than just reducing hypertension, and people started using it to treat obesity, diabetes, cancer, and cardiac disorders.

To study the impact of sodium intake, a scientist used three experimental groups. Each group was assigned a diet with varying sodium levels. One was to take 3300 mg sodium per day; the second had to use 2300 mg per day, and the third one was put on a diet having 1500 mg sodium per day, about two-thirds of a teaspoon of salt. By restricting the sodium content, all participants showed decreased blood pressure. But the group with the least amount of sodium intake showed the most alleviation in the blood pressure levels. Thus, it was identified that 1500 mg of sodium per day is the threshold amount to maintain blood pressure.

Health Advantages of the DASH Diet

Besides hypertension, there are several health advantages that later came to light as experts recorded the conditions people experience after choosing the diet. Here are some of the known benefits of the DASH diet:

Alleviated Blood Pressure

It is the most obvious and direct outcome of this dietary routine as it restricts the sodium intake, which rightly reduces the risks of high blood pressure by keeping the blood consistency to near normal. People with hypertension disorder should restrict sodium intake the most, whereas others should keep the intake as per the described limits, 1500 mg per day.

Maintained Cholesterol Levels

Since a DASH diet promotes greater use of vegetables, fruits, whole grains, beans, and nuts, it can provide enough fiber to regulate our metabolism and digestive functions. Moreover, it promotes only lean meats and no saturated fats, which also helps to maintain cholesterol levels in the body. Such fats have to be replaced with healthy cholesterol fats to keep the heart running.

Weight Maintenance

Weight loss is another primary objective for people on the DASH diet. With a nutritious and clean diet, anyone can lose their excess weight. Moreover, the DASH diet also promotes proper physical exercise every day, which also proves to be significant in reducing obesity. Sometimes, obesity is the result of inflammation or fluid imbalances in the body, and the DASH diet can even cure that through its progressive health approach.

Reduced Risks of Osteoporosis

Osteoporosis is the degeneration of the bones, and there are many factors associated with it; at the base of it is the decrease of calcium and vitamin D in the body. The DASH diet provides ways and meals to fill this deficiency gap and reduce the risks of osteoporosis, especially in women.

Healthier Kidneys

Kidneys are what control the fluid balance of the body with the help of hormones and minerals. So, a smart diet that is designed with the sole purpose of aiding kidney functions can keep them healthy and functioning properly. Excess salt or oxalate intake can cause kidney stones. The DASH diet reduces the chances of these stones from building up in the kidneys.

Protection From Cancer

The DASH diet has been proven effective in preventing people from different types of cancer, like kidney, lung, prostate, esophagus, rectum, and colon cancers. The diet co-joins all the important factors which can fight against cancer and help prevent the development of cancerous cells.

Prevention From Diabetes

The DASH diet is effective in reducing insulin resistance, which is one of the common causes of diabetes in many people. Reduced weight, an active metabolism, maintained body fluids, daily exercises, increased water consumption, a low sodium diet, and a healthy gut or digestive system are all the factors that link the DASH diet with the reduced risks of diabetes in a person.

Improved Mental Health

Mental health is largely dependent on the type of food you eat. Anxiety, depression, and insomnia are all the outcomes of poor health and a bad lifestyle. The entire neural transmission is controlled by the electrolyte balance in the nervous system. With the DASH diet, you can create optimum conditions for efficient brain functions.

Less Risk of Heart Disease

Since the DASH diet is designed to control the varying blood pressure, it saves the heart from the negative impact of high blood pressure and prevents it from different diseases. Constant high blood pressure burdens the heart and causes the weakening of its walls and valves. Such risks are reduced with the help of the DASH diet.

The DASH Dietary Program

It's not just the sodium on which the DASH diet focuses; there are various forms and types of food that it limits. It also places a large emphasis on a certain amount of food per serving. It creates a special place or a box of food for the entire day and limits your daily intake to a value that would maintain a balance in the diet. Such control is hard to attain when you are not following the DASH diet, as the diet prescribes the entire roadmap to better dietary solutions. It is designed to change the ways we see our food and the way we consume it. It mainly works in two ways. First, it controls the quality of the meal, and second, it controls the quantity of the meal. By doing this, you can achieve increased health benefits that no other diet could guarantee. The food is first placed into categories, like fruits, vegetables, whole grains, beans, nuts, meat, or dairy, then you consider the health impact of each category; their share in a single meal or serving is suggested.

Research-Based Benefits of DASH Dieting

The National Institute of Health in the United States carried out early research on the significance of the DASH Diet. Scientists knew the impact of such a diet, but they needed proof to strengthen their claim. So, three different dietary plans were designed to check the impact. The plan with the most fruits, vegetables, beans, and no fat dairy items came out as the most effective in decreasing the diastolic and systolic blood pressures by 3 mmHg and 6 mmHg, respectively. While the DASH diet sets a limitation on certain food items, it also directs a person to controlled caloric intake. It keeps the daily caloric intake between 1600 to 3100. This fact becomes more relevant when there is obesity that has to be dealt with. By passing the Optimal Macronutrient Intake Trial for heart health, the DASH diet set the record of successfully reducing the routine fat intake, preventing all sorts of heart diseases.

It's a Long-Term Solution

Hypertension sufferers cannot always count on medications for long term health stability. No matter how effective the medicines are, they are not free from side effects. A change in diet and lifestyle can give long term treatment along with necessary prevention. Hypertension is not a temporary disorder; once a person has it, they are forever bound by this problem. It is not a matter of days, it's a matter of the rest of their life. That is why only dietary treatment can save the body from high blood pressure and the problems associated with it.

Helps Manage Type 2 Diabetes

To understand the relevance between the DASH diet and diabetes, it is important to look into the root causes of Type 2 Diabetes. High caloric food or increased body weight both make the body resistant to insulin. When you cross off both those factors, it becomes easier to control Type 2 Diabetes. The DASH diet works to manage both these factors. Firstly, through its regulated serving technique and secondly, through reducing obesity. It makes the body more sensitive to insulin; thus, it decreases the possible risks of high blood sugar levels. Moreover, with the dietary balance the DASH diet creates, it sets the bar for carbohydrate consumption, and in the absence of excess carbohydrates, the body can regulate its insulin production and its functions.

Ten Reasons Why the DASH Diet Truly Works

Talking about the DASH diet outside the theory and more in practice reveals more of its efficiency as a diet. Besides excess research and experiments, the true reasons for people looking into this diet are its certain features. It gives the feeling of ease and convenience, which makes the users more comfortable with its rules and regulations. Here are some of the reasons why the DASH

Diet works amazingly:

Easy to Adopt

The broad range of options available under the label of DASH diet makes it more flexible for all. This is the reason that people find it easier to switch to and harness its true health benefits. It makes adaptability easier for its users.

Promotes Exercise

It is most effective than all the other factors because not only does it focus on the food and its intake, but it also duly stresses daily exercises and routine physical activities. This is the reason why it produces quick, visible results.

All Inclusive

With few limitations, this Diet has taken every food item into its fold with certain modifications. It rightly guides us about the Dos and Don'ts of all the ingredients and prevents us from consuming those which are harmful to the body and its health.

A Well Balanced Approach

One of its biggest advantages is that it maintains balance in our diet, in our routine, our caloric intake, and our nutrition.

Good Caloric Check

Every meal we plan on the DASH diet is pre-calculated in terms of calories. We can easily keep track of the daily caloric intake and consequently restrict them easily by cutting off certain food items.

Prohibits Bad Food

The DASH diet suggests the use of more organic and fresh food and discourages the use of processed food and junk items available in stores. So, it creates better eating habits for the users.

Focused on Prevention

Though it is proven to be a cure for many diseases, it is described as more of a preventive strategy.

Slow Yet Progressive Changes

The diet is not highly restrictive and accommodates gradual changes towards achieving the ultimate health goal. You can set up your daily, weekly, or even monthly goals at your own convenience.

Long Term Effects

The results of the DASH diet are not just incredible, but they are also long-lasting. It is considered slow in progress, but the effects last longer.

Accelerates Metabolism

With its healthy approach to life, the DASH diet has the ability to activate our metabolism and boost it for better functioning of the body.

CHAPTER 2:

Breakfast & Smoothies

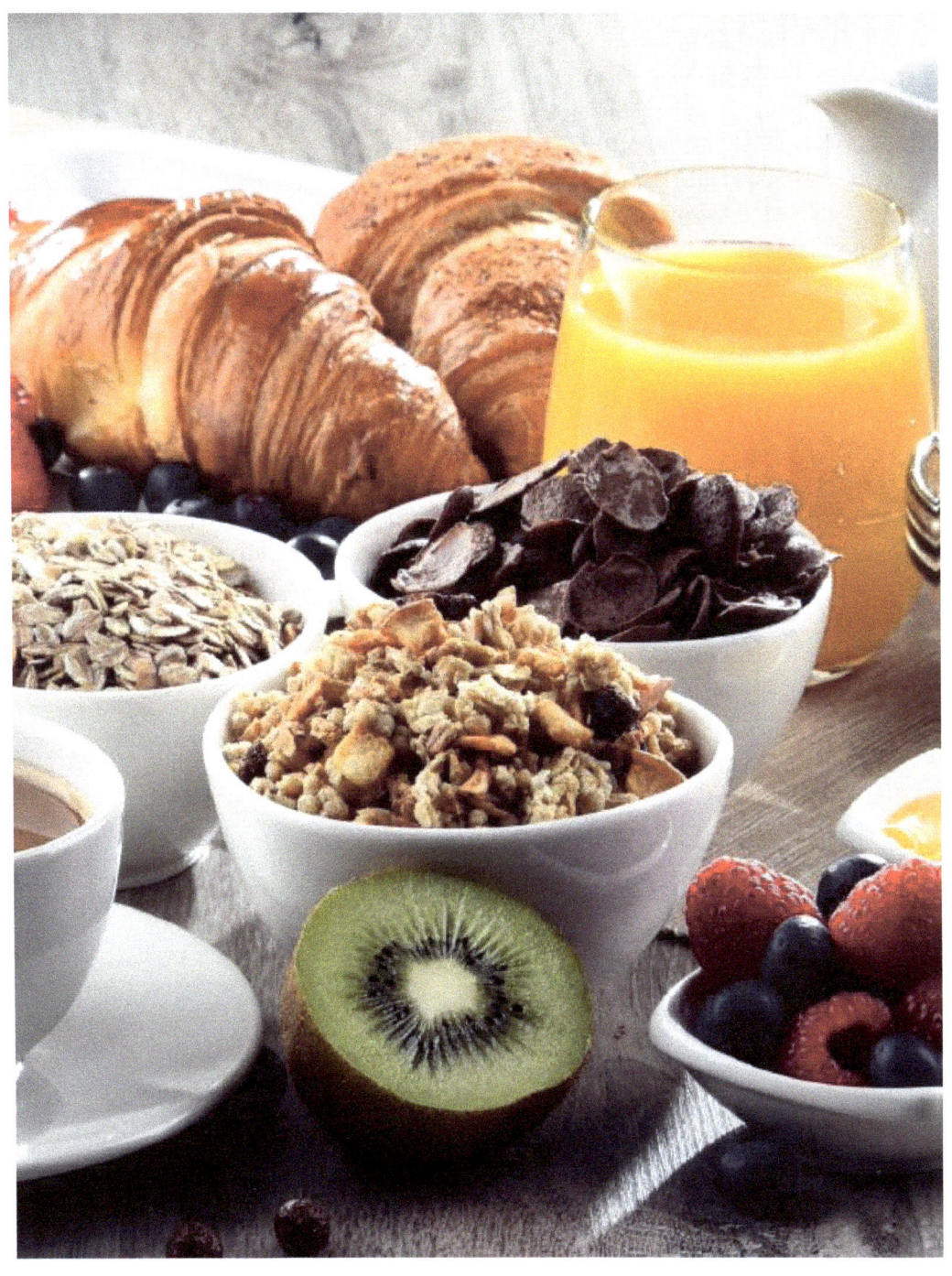

Yogurt & Banana Muffins

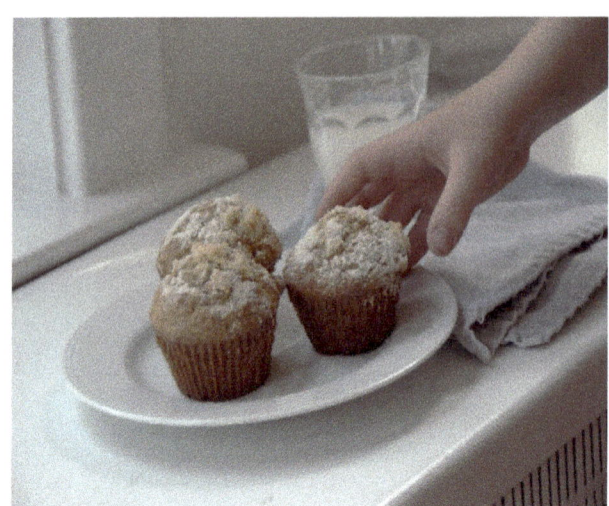

Preparation Time: 15 minutes

Cooking Time: 25 minutes

Servings: 2

Ingredients:

- 3 bananas, large & mashed
- 1 teaspoon baking soda
- 1 cup old fashioned rolled oats
- 2 tablespoons flaxseed, ground
- 1 cup whole wheat flour
- ¼ cup applesauce, unsweetened
- ½ cup plain yogurt
- ¼ cup brown sugar
- 2 teaspoons vanilla extract, pure

Directions:

1. Start by turning the oven to 355, and then get out a muffin tray. Grease it and then get out a bowl.
2. Mix your flaxseed, oats, soda, and flour in a bowl.
3. Mash your banana and then mix in your sugar, vanilla, yogurt, and applesauce. Stir in your oats mixture, making sure it's well combined. It's okay for it to be lumpy.
4. Divide between muffin trays, and then bake for twenty-five minutes. Serve warm.

Nutrition:

- Calories: 316
- Protein: 11.2 g
- Fat: 14.5 g
- Carbs: 36.8 g
- Sodium: 469 mg
- Cholesterol: 43 mg

Berry Quinoa Bowls

Preparation Time: 15 minutes

Cooking Time: 20 minutes

Servings: 2

Ingredients:

- 1 small peach, sliced
- 2/3 + ¾ cup milk, low fat
- 1/3 cup uncooked quinoa, rinsed well
- ½ teaspoon vanilla extract, pure
- 2 teaspoons brown sugar
- 14 blueberries
- 2 teaspoons honey, raw
- 12 raspberries

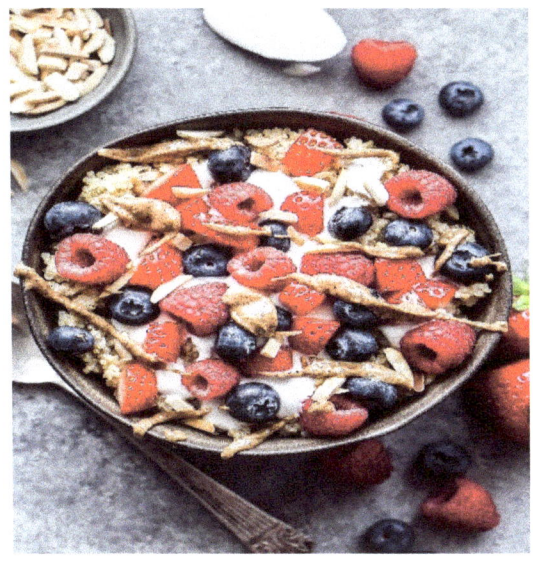

Directions:

1. Start to boil your quinoa, vanilla, 2/3 cup milk, and brown sugar together for five minutes before reducing it to a simmer. Cook for twenty minutes.
2. Heat a grill pan that's been greased over medium heat, and then add in your peaches to grill for one minute per side.
3. Heat the remaining ¾ cup of milk in your microwave. Cook the quinoa with a splash of milk, berries, and grilled peaches. Don't forget to drizzle with honey before serving it.

Nutrition:

- Calories: 435
- Protein: 9.2 g
- Fat: 13.7 g
- Carbs: 24.9 g
- Sodium: 141 mg
- Cholesterol: 78 mg

Pineapple Green Smoothie

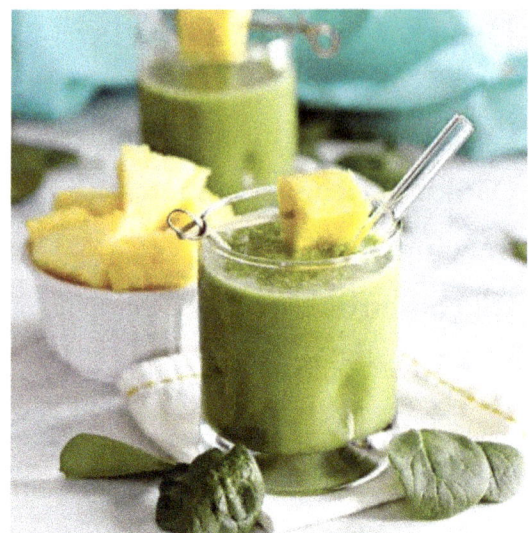

Preparation Time: 5 minutes

Cooking Time: 0 minutes

Servings: 2

Ingredients:

- 1 ¼ cups orange juice
- ½ cup Greek yogurt, plain
- 1 cup spinach, fresh
- 1 cup pineapple, frozen & chunked
- 1 cup mango, frozen & chunked
- 1 tablespoon ground flaxseed
- 1 teaspoon granulated stevia

Directions:

1. Start by blending everything together until smooth, and then serve cold.

Nutrition:

- Calories: 213
- Protein: 9 g
- Fat: 2 g
- Carbs: 43 g
- Sodium: 44 mg
- Cholesterol: 2.5 mg

Peanut Butter & Banana Smoothie

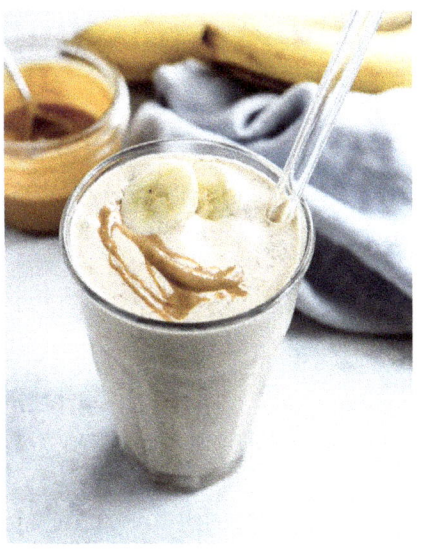

Preparation Time: 5 minutes

Cooking Time: 0 minutes

Servings: 1

Ingredients:

- 1 cup milk, nonfat
- 1 tablespoon peanut butter, all natural
- 1 banana, frozen & sliced

Directions:

1. Start by blending everything together until smooth.

Nutrition:

- Calories: 146
- Protein: 1.1 g
- Fat: 5.5 g
- Carbs: 1.8 g
- Sodium: 40 mg

Pumpkin-Hazelnut Tea Cake

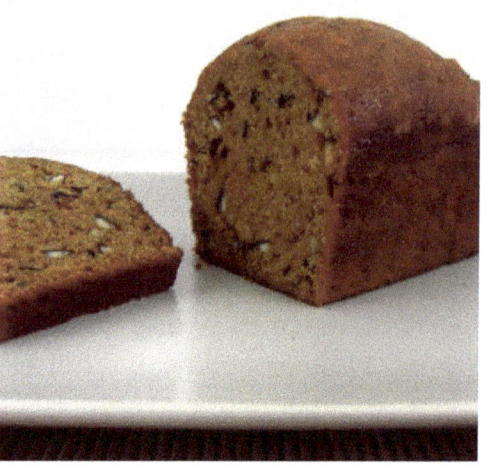

Preparation Time: 5 minutes

Cooking Time: 55 minutes

Servings: 2

Ingredients:

- 3 tablespoons canola oil
- 3/4 cup homemade or unsweetened canned pumpkin puree
- 1/2 cup honey
- 3 tablespoons firmly packed brown sugar
- 2 eggs, lightly beaten
- 1 cup whole-wheat (whole-meal) flour
- 1/2 cup all-purpose (plain) flour
- 2 tablespoons flaxseed
- 1/2 teaspoon baking powder
- 1/2 teaspoon ground allspice
- 1/2 teaspoon ground cinnamon
- 1/2 teaspoon ground nutmeg
- 1/4 teaspoon ground cloves
- 1/4 teaspoon salt
- 2 tablespoons chopped hazelnuts (filberts)

Directions:

1. Grease an 8x4 inch loaf pan with cooking spray. Set the oven to 350 degrees F.
2. Beat pumpkin puree with brown sugar, honey, eggs, and canola oil in a mixer.
3. Stir in flaxseed, allspice, baking powder, flours, cinnamon, cloves, salt, flours, and salt.
4. Mix well until it forms a smooth batter, transfer this batter to the loaf pan. Top it evenly with hazelnuts.
5. Press the nuts down, then bake for 55 minutes.
6. Allow the bread to cool for 10 minutes.
7. Slice and serve.

Nutrition:

- Calories 166
- Total Fat 6.5 g
- Cholesterol 43 mg
- Sodium 469 mg
- Total Carbs 27.8 g
- Protein 11.2 g

Raspberry Chocolate Scones

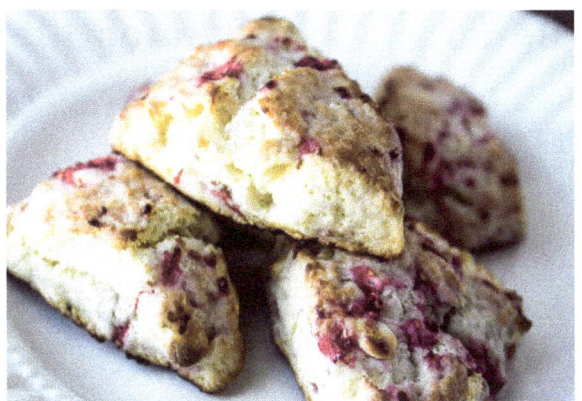

Preparation Time: 7 minutes

Cooking Time: 12 minutes

Servings: 2

Ingredients:

- 1 cup whole-wheat pastry flour
- 1 cup all-purpose flour
- 1 tablespoon baking powder
- 1/4 teaspoon baking soda
- 1/3 cup trans-fat-free buttery spread
- 1/2 cup fresh or frozen raspberries
- 1/4 cup miniature chocolate chips
- 1 cup plus 2 tablespoons plain fat-free yogurt
- 2 tablespoons honey
- 1/2 teaspoon sugar
- 1/4 teaspoon cinnamon

Directions:

1. Preheat the oven to 400 degrees F.
2. Combine flours with baking soda and baking powder in a mixing bowl.
3. Cut the butter into the dry mixture until it forms a crumbly mixture.
4. Fold in chocolate chips and berries.
5. Pour in honey and yogurt, then stir the mixture gently to form a crumbly batter.
6. Knead the dough ball on a surface, then spread it into ½ inch thick circle.
7. Slice the sheet into 12 wedges, then arrange them on a greased baking tray.
8. Sprinkle sugar and cinnamon mixture on top.
9. Bake them for 12 minutes at 400 degrees F.
10. Serve and enjoy.

Nutrition:

- Calories 149
- Total Fat 13.7 g
- Cholesterol 78 mg
- Sodium 141 mg
- Total Carbs 22.9 g
- Fiber 3.2 g
- Sugar 1.3 g
- Protein 4.2 g

Banana Almond Smoothie

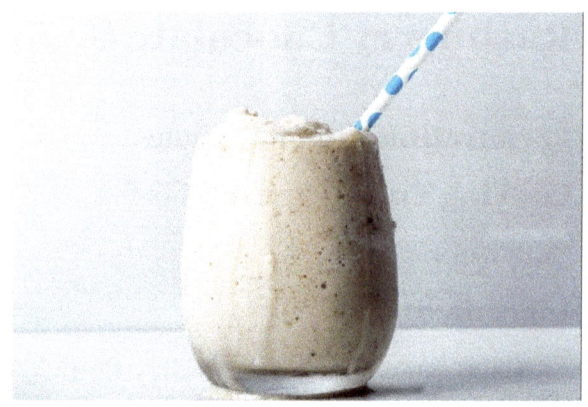

Preparation Time: 3 minutes

Cooking Time: 0 minutes

Servings: 2

Ingredients:

- 10 ounces (2 large) banana, frozen
- 4 tablespoons flaxseeds
- 2 tablespoons almond butter
- 1 cup almond milk
- ½ teaspoon honey
- ¼ teaspoon vanilla extract

Directions:

1. Using a blender, combine all the ingredients, until it becomes smooth.
2. Transfer the entire mix into two serving glass.
3. Serve fresh or refrigerate and consume.

Nutrition:

- Calories: 581
- Total Fat: 42.5 g
- Total Carbs: 47.5 g
- Dietary Fiber 11.7 g
- Cholesterol: 0 mg
- Sodium: 25 mg
- Protein: 10.3 g

Blueberry Banana Muffins

Preparation Time: 20 minutes

Cooking Time: 25 minutes

Serving: 2

Ingredients:

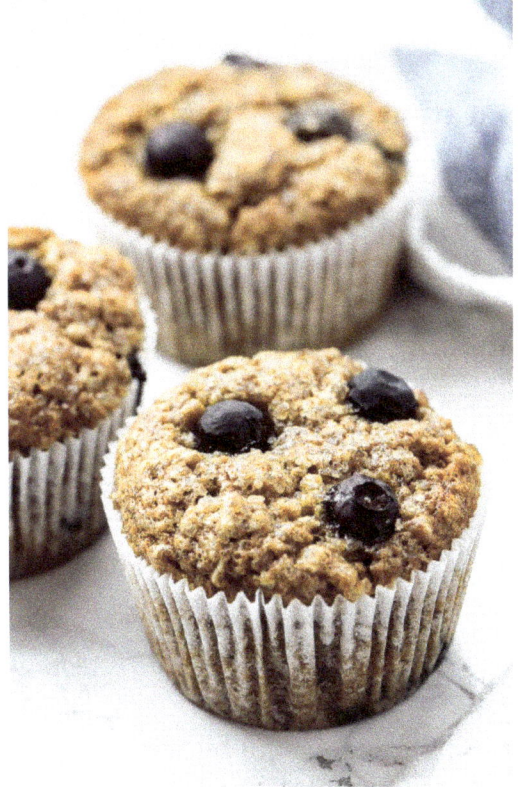

- 20 ounces (4 large) ripe banana, mashed
- 1¼ cups blueberries, fresh or frozen
- ¾ cup+2 tablespoons almond milk, unsweetened
- ¼ cup maple syrup
- 1 teaspoon apple cider vinegar
- 1 teaspoon vanilla extract
- 2 cups white flour
- ¼ cup coconut oil
- 2 teaspoons baking powder
- 6 tablespoons cane sugar
- 1½ teaspoons cinnamon, ground
- ½ teaspoon baking soda
- ½ teaspoon salt - ½ cup walnut halves, chopped

Directions:

1. Set the oven to 360°F and preheat. Spray some cooking oil into the muffin tin.
2. In a standard-sized bowl, mash all bananas and take ¾ cup. Refrigerate the remaining portion for making the smoothie. Put the mashed banana into a bowl along with the vinegar, milk, maple syrup, and vanilla. Do not stir. In a big bowl, mix all the dry ingredients like sugar, flour, cinnamon, baking powder, salt, and baking soda.
3. Stir in coconut oil into the dry mixture and combine well.
4. Pour all wet items mentioned in step 4 on top of the dry ingredients and blend them. Avoid over mixing. Put walnuts into the mix and after that the blueberries, and make sure that you have not over mix the ingredients. Over mixing may make it like a thick batter and the muffin become strong and spoil the dish. Spoon ¼ cup of batter into every tin of muffin, Bake the muffin at 370°F for 22 to 27 minutes. Insert a toothpick to check its baking status. When inserted the toothpick, it should come out clean. After baking is over, keep it 5-8 minutes to settle down and transfer to the cooling rack, keep it there for 15 minutes. Serve fresh.

Nutrition:

- Calories: 296 Total Carbohydrates: 36.3 g Dietary Fiber: 1.7 g Sugars: 16.4 g
- Total Fat: 14.6 g Cholesterol: 0 mg Sodium: 161 mg Protein: 3.9 g

Easy Buckwheat Crepes

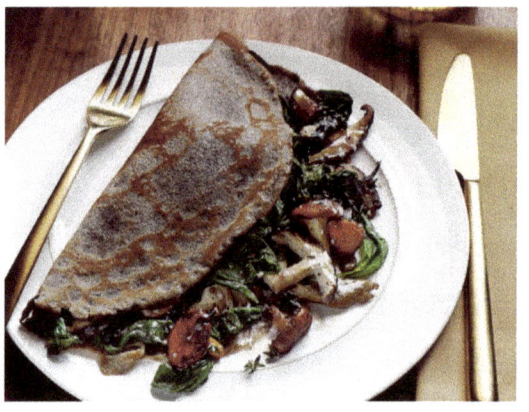

Preparation Time: 10 minutes

Cooking Time: 15 minutes

Serving: 2

Ingredients:

For making Crepes:

- 1 cup buckwheat flour, raw, un-toasted
- 1¾ cups light coconut milk, low-fat
- ¾ tablespoon flaxseed
- 1 tablespoon melted coconut oil
- ⅛ teaspoon ground cinnamon
- ⅛ teaspoon salt
- ⅛ teaspoon stevia

For fillings:

- 8 tablespoons nut butter
- 6 tablespoons granola
- 6 tablespoons compote
- 8 tablespoons -coconut whipped cream
- 3 cinnamon baked apples

Directions:

1. Put buckwheat flour, flaxseed, light coconut milk, coconut oil, salt, cinnamon, and stevia into a blender. Blend the above ingredients until it combines well. Blend until it turns into a pourable batter. Add a little buckwheat flour if the dough is too thin. If the batter is too thick, add some dairy-free milk.
2. Heat a nonstick skillet on medium temperature. Once, the skillet is hot, spread some oil in the bottom evenly. When the oiled surface of the skillet becomes hot, pour ¼ cup of batter into the skillet and cook until the top turns bubbly and the edges become dry. Carefully flip the crepes to cook for 2 minutes more. Do not let the skillet become too hot. Repeat the process until you finish all the crepes. To keep the warmness of the crepes, keep parchment paper between the crepes.
3. Serve it with vegan butter, or maple syrup or nut butter, or coconut whipped cream or cinnamon banked apples. You can also serve it with bananas or berries.
4. It's best if you serve it fresh, but you can easily store leftovers sealed in the refrigerator for up to 3 days. You can use it after reheating.

Nutrition:

- Calories: 230 Total Fat: 16.6 g Total Carbs: 24.6 g Dietary Fiber: 3.2 g
- Total Sugars: 3 g Cholesterol: 0 mg Sodium: 39 mg Protein: 4.2 g

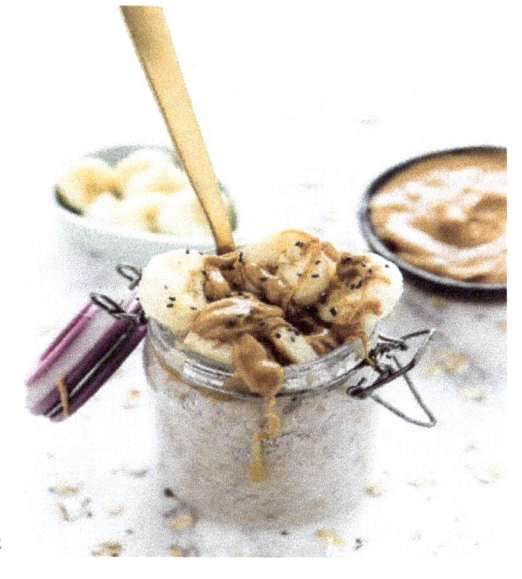

Peanut Butter Oats in the Jar

Preparation Time: 6 hours and 5 minutes

Cooking Time: 0 minutes

Servings: 1

Ingredients

For the oats:

- ½ cup gluten-free rolled oats
- ½ cup unsweetened, plain almond milk
- 4 tablespoons natural salted peanut butter
- 1 tablespoon maple syrup (or stevia, organic brown sugar)
- ¾ tablespoon chia seeds

For the toppings (optional):

- Banana, sliced
- Strawberries or raspberries
- Chia seeds

Directions:

1. Combine the almond milk, peanut butter, chia seeds, and maple syrup in a Mason jar. Stir but don't over-mix to leave swirls of peanut butter. Add the oats and stir again.
2. Press down the oats with a spoon to make sure they are soaked in the milk mixture.
3. Secure the jar with a lid and refrigerate for at least 6 hours.
4. To serve, garnish with toppings of choice.

Note: Nutritional info does not include toppings.

Nutrition:

- Calories: 454
- Carbohydrates: 50.9g
- Fat: 3.9g
- Fiber: 12g
- Protein: 14.6g
- Sodium: 162mg
- Sugar: 14.9g

Fruit Smoothie

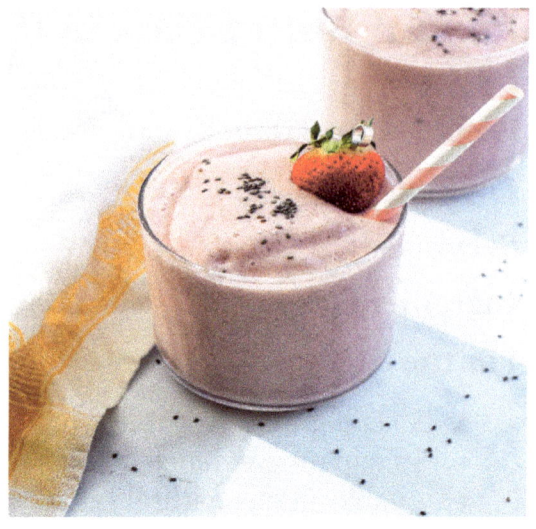

Preparation Time: 5 minutes

Cooking Time: 5 minutes

Servings: 1

Ingredients:

- One-fourth cup blueberries
- Four oz. strawberries
- One-half orange, peeled
- Four oz. papaya peeled, seeded, and diced
- One-fourth cup ice cubes
- Four oz. soy milk

Directions:

1. Pulse the blueberries, strawberries, peeled orange, and milk in a blender for approximately half a minute.
2. Combine the ice cubes and papaya and continue to blend for another 30 seconds.
3. Transfer to a glass and enjoy immediately.
4. You can also use frozen fruit if you prefer.

Nutrition:

- Sodium: 71 mg
- Protein: 6 g
- Fat: 3 g
- Sugar: 26 g
- Calories: 184
- Carbs: 43 g

Green Smoothie

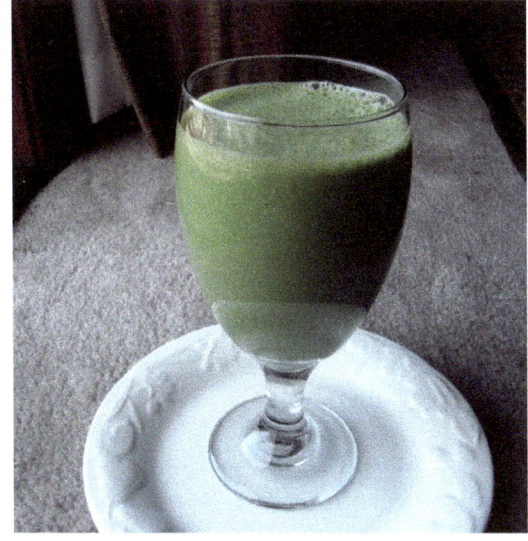

Preparation Time: 5 minutes

Cooking Time: 5 minutes

Servings: 1

Ingredients:

- One-fourth cup yogurt, non-fat and plain
- One-half tsp. vanilla extract
- One cup spinach
- One medium banana
- One-half cup milk, fat-free
- Three-fourths cup mango
- One-fourth cup whole oats

Directions:

1. Using a blender, combine the baby spinach, yogurt, whole oats, milk, and mango. Pulse for approximately half a minute.
2. Blend the banana and vanilla extract and pulse for an additional half minute until smooth.
3. Empty into a serving glass and enjoy immediately.

Nutrition:

- Sodium: 20 mg
- Protein: 2 g
- Fat: 0 g
- Sugar: 5 g
- Calories: 48
- Carbs: 38 g

Heart-Friendly Sweet Potato-Oats Waffles

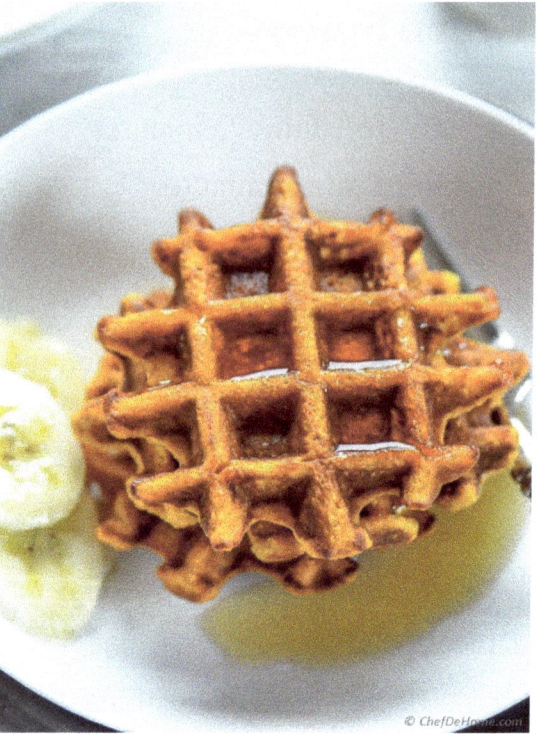

Preparation Time: 5 minutes

Cooking Time: 10 minutes

Servings: 2

Ingredients:

For the waffles:

- 1 cup rolled oats
- ½ cup Sweet potato, cooked and skin removed
- 1 whole egg
- 1 egg white
- 1 cup almond milk
- 1 tablespoon honey
- 1 tablespoon olive oil
- ¼ teaspoon baking powder
- ¼ teaspoon salt

To serve:

- Banana, sliced
- Maple syrup

Directions:

1. Preheat the waffle iron.
2. Meanwhile, add all the ingredients to a blender and process until pureed. Let the mixture rest for 10 minutes.
3. Coat the waffle iron with a nonstick cooking spray.
4. Pour ⅓ cup of the batter into each mold. Cook about 3-4 minutes per batch or 30 seconds longer after the light indicator turns green. Usually, waffles are done after the steam stops coming out of the waffle iron.
5. Serve with banana slices and maple syrup on top.

Nutrition:

- Calories: 287 Carbohydrates: 54g
- Fat: 8.39g Fiber: 7.2g
- Protein: 12.42g
- Sodium: 285mg
- Sugar: 22g

Rhubarb Pecan Muffins

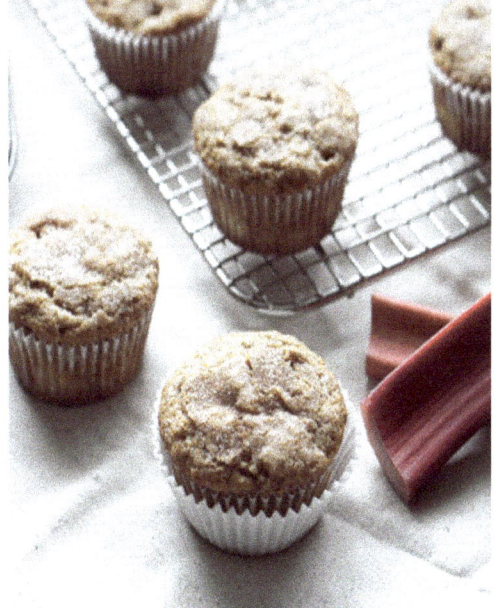

Preparation Time: 10 minutes

Cooking Time: 30 minutes

Servings: 2

Ingredients:

- 1 cup all-purpose (plain) flour
- 1 cup whole-wheat (whole-meal) flour
- 1/2 cup sugar
- 1 1/2 teaspoon baking powder
- 1/2 teaspoon baking soda
- 1/2 teaspoon salt
- 2 egg whites
- 2 tablespoons canola oil
- 2 tablespoons unsweetened applesauce
- 2 teaspoons grated orange peel
- 3/4 cup calcium-fortified orange juice
- 1 1/4 cup finely chopped rhubarb
- 2 tablespoons chopped pecans

Directions:

1. Set the oven to heat at 350 degrees F. Layer a muffin pan with muffin paper.
2. Combine flours with baking soda, baking powder, sugar, and salt in a bowl.
3. Whisk egg whites with orange peel, orange juice, applesauce, and canola oil in another container.
4. Add this wet mixture to the dry ingredients and mix well until smooth.
5. Fold in chopped rhubarb, then divide the mixture into the muffin cups.
6. Top the batter with a ½ teaspoon with chopped pecans.
7. Bake the muffin for 30 minutes then allow them to cool.
8. Serve.

Nutrition:

- Calories 143
- Total Fat 15.5 g
- Cholesterol 0 mg
- Sodium 31 mg
- Total Carbs 21.8 g
- Fiber 2.6 g
- Sugar 4.5 g
- Protein 4.1 g

Whole-Wheat Pretzels

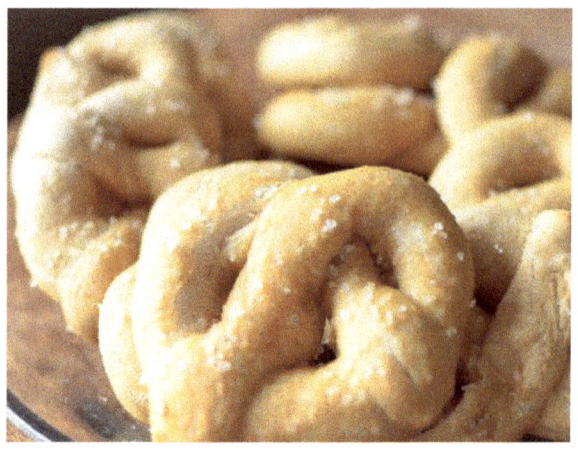

Preparation Time: 10 minutes

Cooking Time: 15 minutes

Servings: 2

Ingredients:

- 1 package active dry yeast
- 2 teaspoons brown sugar
- 1/2 teaspoon kosher salt
- 1 1/2 cups warm water
- 1 cup bread flour
- 3 cups whole-wheat flour
- 1 tablespoon olive oil
- 1/2 cup wheat gluten
- Cooking spray, as needed
- 1/4 cup baking soda
- 1 egg white or 1/4 cup egg substitute
- 1 tablespoon of sesame, poppy, or sunflower seeds

Directions:

1. Preheat the oven to 450 degrees F.
2. Mix yeast with salt, sugar, and water in a bowl and let it rest for 5 minutes.
3. Combine flours with gluten and olive oil in a processor.
4. Mix in the yeast mixture and knead the dough until smooth.
5. Cover the dough in the bowl with a plastic sheet and keep it in a warm place for 1 hour until the dough has raised.
6. Now, punch down the dough and divide the dough into 14 pieces.
7. Roll each piece into long ropes and make a pretzel shape out of this dough rope.
8. Boil 10 cups of water with ¼ cup baking soda in a pot. Place the pretzels in the water.
9. Cook each pretzel for 30 seconds then immediately transfer them to a baking pan lined with parchment paper using a slotted spoon.
10. Brush each pretzel with whisked egg whites and drizzle sesame, sunflower, and poppy seeds on top.
11. Bake them for 15 minutes at 450 degrees F
12. Serve.

Nutrition:

- Calories 148 Total Fat 12.8 g
- Cholesterol 112 mg Sodium 32 mg
- Total Carbs 31.5 g Fiber 4.2 g Sugar 2.5 g Protein 7.6 g

Mushroom Frittata

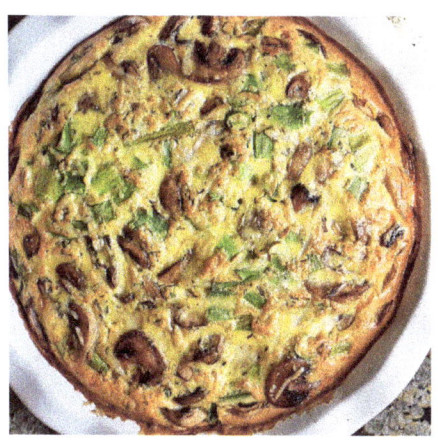

Preparation Time: 15 minutes

Cooking Time: 10 minutes

Servings: 2

Ingredients:

- 4 shallots, chopped
- 1 tablespoons butter
- 2 teaspoons parsley, fresh & diced
- ½ lb. mushrooms, fresh & diced
- 3 eggs
- 1 teaspoon thyme
- 5 egg whites
- ¼ teaspoon black pepper
- 1 tablespoon half & half, fat-free
- ¼ cup parmesan cheese, grated

Directions:

1. Start by turning the oven to 350, and then get out a skillet. Grease it with butter, letting it melt over medium heat.
2. Once your butter is hot adding in your shallots. Cook until golden brown, which should take roughly five minutes.
3. Stir in your thyme, pepper, parsley, and mushrooms.
4. Beat your eggs, egg whites, parmesan, and half and half together in a bowl.
5. Pour the mixture over your mushrooms, cooking for two minutes. Transfer the skillet to the oven, and bake for fifteen minutes. Slice to serve warm.

Nutrition:

- Calories: 391
- Protein: 7.6 g
- Fat: 12.8 g
- Carbs: 31.5 g
- Sodium: 32 mg
- Cholesterol: 112 mg

Cheesy Omelet

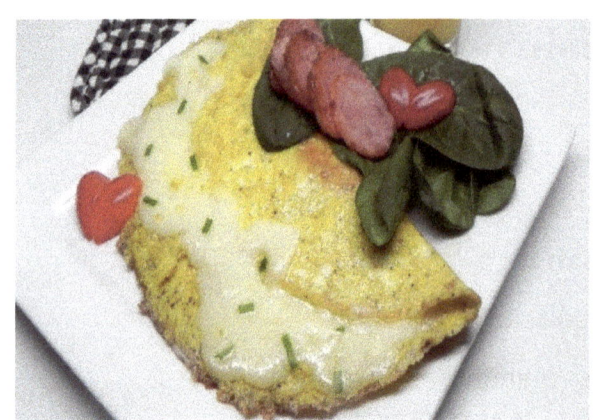

Preparation Time: 10 minutes

Cooking Time: 10 minutes

Servings: 2

Ingredients:

- 4 eggs
- 4 cups broccoli florets
- 1 tablespoon olive oil
- 1 cup egg whites
- ¼ cup cheddar, reduced-fat
- ¼ cup romano, grated
- ¼ teaspoon sea salt, fine
- ¼ teaspoon black pepper
- Cooking spray as needed

Directions:

1. Start by heating your oven to 350, and then steam your broccoli over boiling water for five to seven minutes. It should be tender.
2. Mash the broccoli into small pieces, and then toss with salt, pepper, and olive oil.
3. Get out a muffin tray and then grease it with cooking spray. Divide your broccoli between the cups, and then get out a bowl.
4. In the bowl beat your eggs with salt, pepper, egg whites, and parmesan.
5. Pour your batter over the broccoli, and then top with cheese. Bake for two minutes before serving warm.

Nutrition:

- Calories: 427
- Protein: 7.5 g
- Fat: 8.6 g
- Carbs: 13 g
- Sodium: 282 mg
- Cholesterol: 4.2 g

Ginger Congee

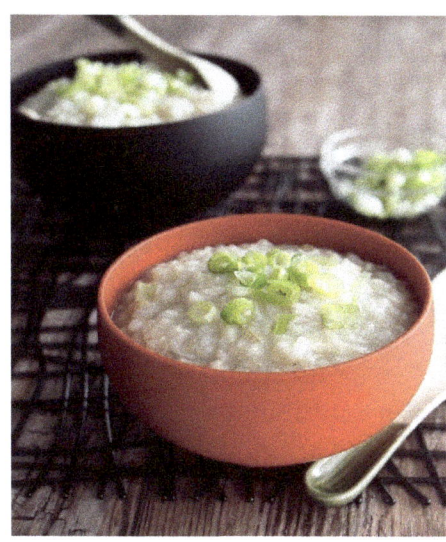

Preparation Time: 10 minutes

Cooking Time: 1 hour

Servings: 1

Ingredients:

- 1 cup white rice, long grain & rinsed
- 7 cups chicken stock
- 1 inch ginger, peeled & sliced thin
- green onion, sliced for garnish
- sesame seed oil to garnish

Directions:

1. Start by boiling your ginger, rice, and salt in a pot. Allow it to simmer and reduce to low heat. Give it a gentle stir, and then allow it to cook for an hour. It should be thick and creamy.
2. Garnish by drizzling with sesame oil and serving warm.

Nutrition:

- Calories: 510
- Protein: 13.5 g
- Carbs: 60.7 g
- Fat: 24.7 g
- Sodium: 840 mg
- Cholesterol: 0 mg

Egg Melts

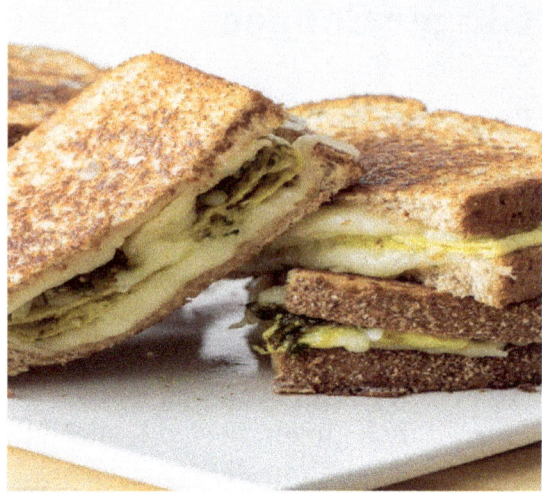

Preparation Time: 10 minutes

Cooking Time: 10 minutes

Servings: 2

Ingredients:

- 1 teaspoon olive oil
- 2 English muffins, whole grain & split
- 4 scallions, sliced fine
- 8 egg whites, whisked
- ¼ teaspoon sea salt, fine
- ¼ teaspoon black pepper
- ½ cup Swiss cheese, shredded & reduced fat
- ½ cup grape tomatoes, quartered

Directions:

1. Set the oven to broil, and then put your English muffins on a baking sheet. Make sure the split side is facing up. Broil for two minutes. They should turn golden around the edges.
2. Get out a skillet and grease with oil. Place it over medium heat, and cook your scallions for three minutes.
3. Beat your egg whites with salt and pepper, and pour this over your scallions.
4. Cook for another minute, stirring gently.
5. Spread this on your muffins, and top with remaining scallions if desired, cheese and tomatoes. Broil for 1 and a half more minutes to melt the cheese and serve warm.

Nutrition:

- Calories: 212
- Protein: 5.3 g
- Fat: 3.9 g
- Carbs: 14.3 g
- Sodium: 135 mg
- Cholesterol: 0 mg

CHAPTER 3:

Salads

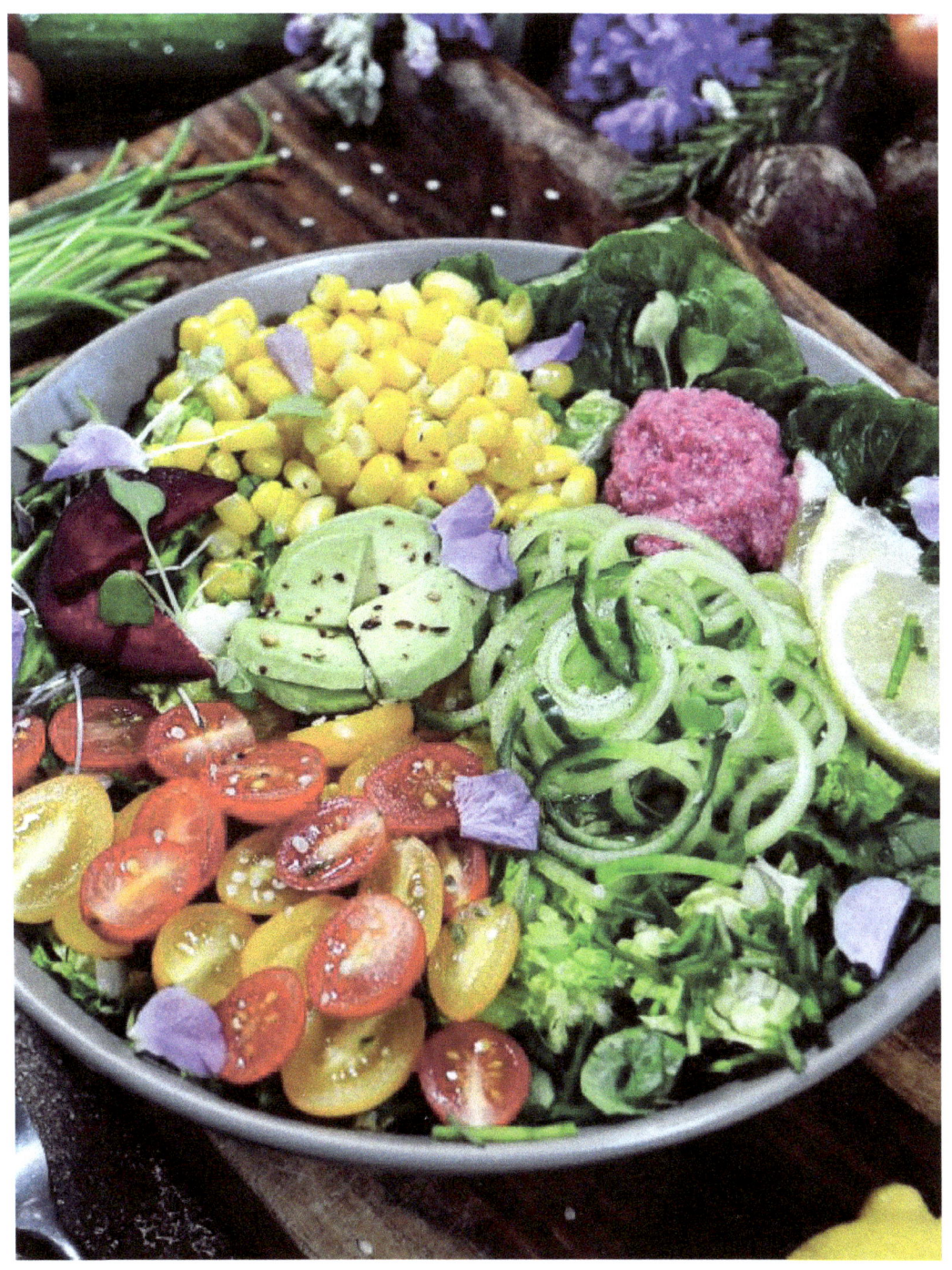

Spring Greens Salad

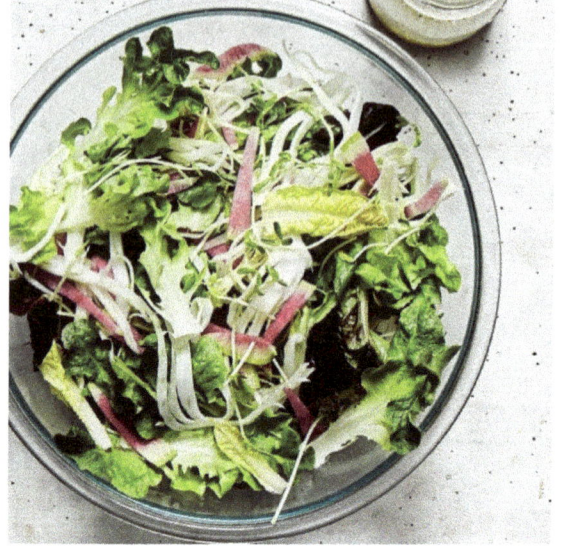

Preparation Time: 5 minutes

Cooking Time: 0 minutes

Servings: 2

Ingredients:

- ½ cup radish, sliced
- 1 cup fresh spinach, chopped
- ½ cup green peas, cooked
- ½ lemon
- 1 cup arugula, chopped
- 1 tablespoon avocado oil
- ½ teaspoon dried sage

Directions:

1. In the salad bowl, mix up radish, spinach, green peas, arugula, and dried sage.
2. Then squeeze the lemon over the salad.
3. Add avocado oil and shake the salad.

Nutrition:

- 54 calories
- 3.1g protein
- 9g carbohydrates
- 1.3g fat
- 3.6g fiber
- 0 mg cholesterol

Tuna Salad

Preparation Time: 7 minutes

Cooking Time: 0 minutes

Servings: 2

Ingredients:

- ½ cup low-fat Greek yogurt
- 8 oz tuna, canned
- ½ cup fresh parsley, chopped
- 1 cup corn kernels, cooked
- ½ teaspoon ground black pepper

Directions:

1. Mix up tuna, parsley, kernels, and ground black pepper.
2. Then add yogurt and stir the salad until it is homogenous.

Nutrition:

- 172 calories
- 17.8g protein
- 13.6g carbohydrates
- 5.5g fat
- 1.4g fiber
- 19mg cholesterol
- 55mg sodium

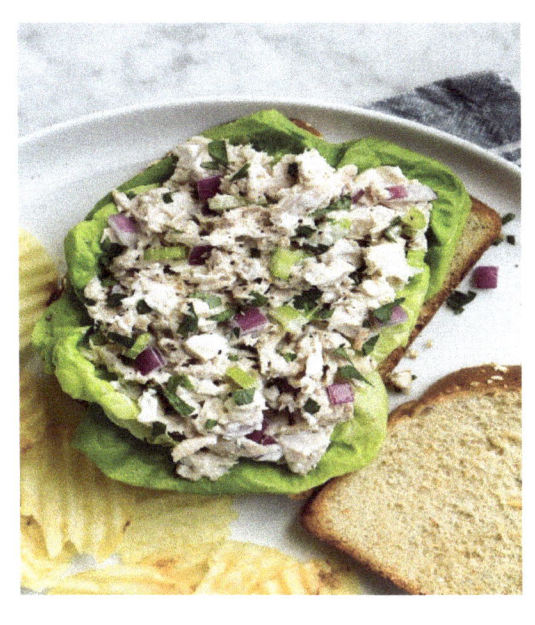

Fish Salad

Preparation Time: 5 minutes

Cooking Time: 0 minutes

Servings: 2

Ingredients:

- 7 oz canned salmon, shredded
- 1 tablespoon lime juice
- 1 tablespoon low-fat yogurt
- 1 cup baby spinach, chopped
- 1 teaspoon capers, drained and chopped

Directions:

1. Mix up all ingredients together and transfer them into the salad bowl.

Nutrition:

- 71 calories
- 10.1g protein
- 0.8g carbohydrates
- 3.2g fat
- 0.2g fiber
- 22mg cholesterol
- 52mg sodium

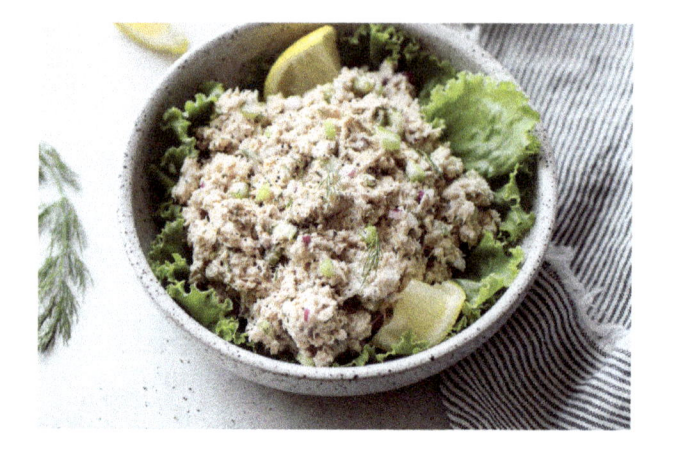

Salmon Salad

Preparation Time: 10 minutes

Cooking Time: 0 minutes

Servings: 2

Ingredients:

- 4 oz canned salmon, flaked
- 1 tablespoon lemon juice
- 2 tablespoons red bell pepper, chopped
- 1 tablespoon red onion, chopped
- 1 teaspoon dill, chopped
- 1 tablespoon olive oil

Directions:

1. Mix up all ingredients in the salad bowl.

Nutrition:

- 119 calories
- 8.3g protein
- 6.6g carbohydrates
- 7.3g fat
- 1.2g fiber
- 17mg cholesterol
- 21mg sodium

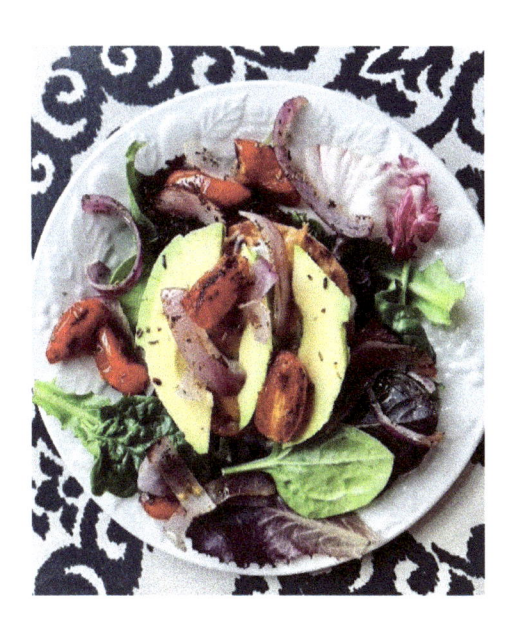

Arugula Salad with Shallot

Preparation Time: 10 minutes

Cooking Time: 0 minutes

Servings: 2

Ingredients:

- 1 cup cucumber, chopped
- 1 tablespoon lemon juice
- 1 tablespoon avocado oil
- 2 shallots, chopped
- ½ cup black olives, sliced
- 3 cups arugula, chopped

Directions:

1. Mix up all ingredients from the list above in the salad bowl and refrigerate in the fridge for 5 minutes.

Nutrition:

- 33 calories
- 0.8g protein
- 2.9g carbohydrates
- 2.4g fat
- 1.1g fiber
- 0mg cholesterol
- 152mg sodium

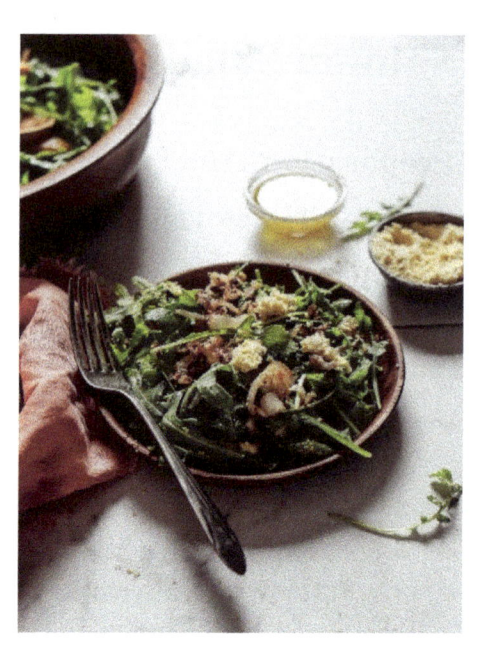

Watercress Salad

Preparation Time: 10 minutes

Cooking Time: 4 minutes

Servings: 2

Ingredients:

- 2 cups asparagus, chopped
- 16 ounces shrimp, cooked
- 4 cups watercress, torn
- 1 tablespoon apple cider vinegar
- ¼ cup olive oil

Directions:

1. In the mixing bowl mix up asparagus, shrimps, watercress, and olive oil.

Nutrition:

- 264 calories
- 28.3g protein
- 4.5g carbohydrates
- 14.8g fat
- 1.8g fiber
- 239mg cholesterol
- 300mg sodium

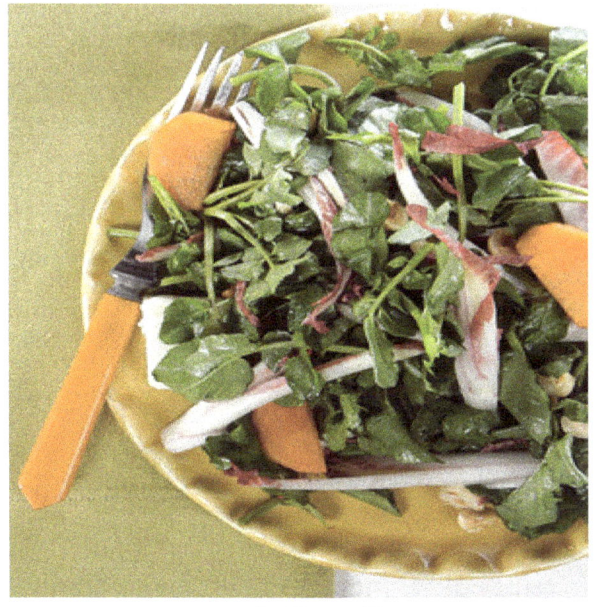

Seafood Arugula Salad

Preparation Time: 5 minutes

Cooking Time: 10 minutes

Servings: 2

Ingredients:

- 1 tablespoon olive oil
- 2 cups shrimps, cooked
- 1 cup arugula
- 1 tablespoon cilantro, chopped

Directions:

1. Put all ingredients in the salad bowl and shake well.

Nutrition:

- 61 calories
- 6.6g protein
- 0.2g carbohydrates
- 3.7g fat
- 0.1g fiber
- 123mg cholesterol
- 216mg sodium

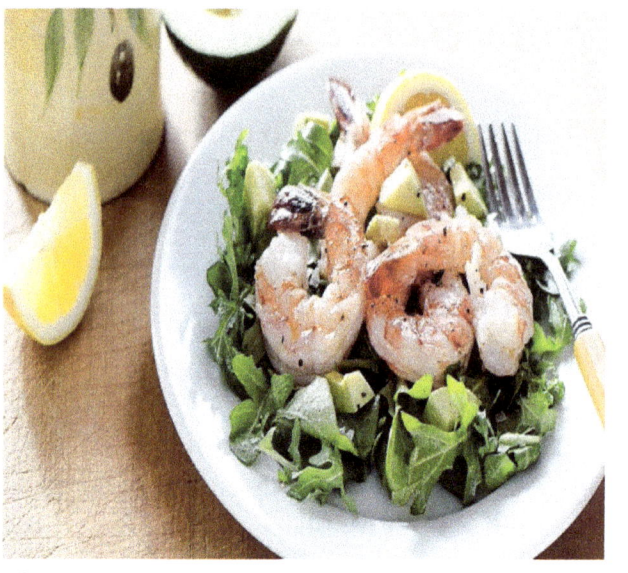

Smoked Salad

Preparation Time: 10 minutes

Cooking Time: 0 minutes

Servings: 2

Ingredients:

- 1 mango, chopped
- 4 cups lettuce, chopped
- 8 oz smoked turkey, chopped
- 2 tablespoons low-fat yogurt
- 1 teaspoon smoked paprika

Directions:

1. Mix up all ingredients in the bowls and transfer them to the serving plates.

Nutrition:

- 88 calories
- 7.1g protein
- 11.2g carbohydrates
- 1.9g fat
- 1.3g fiber
- 25mg cholesterol
- 350mg sodium

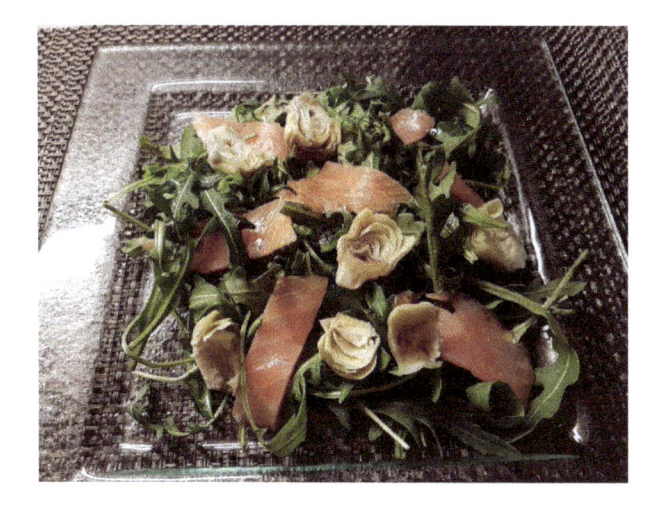

Avocado Salad

Preparation Time: 5 minutes

Cooking Time: 0 minutes

Servings: 2

Ingredients:

- ½ teaspoon ground black pepper
- 1 avocado, peeled, pitted and sliced
- 4 cups lettuce, chopped
- 1 cup black olives, pitted and halved
- 1 cup tomatoes, chopped
- 1 tablespoon olive oil

Directions:

1. Put all ingredients in the salad bowl and mix up well.

Nutrition:

- 197 calories
- 1.9g protein
- 10g carbohydrates
- 17.1g fat
- 5.4g fiber
- 0mg cholesterol
- 301mg sodium

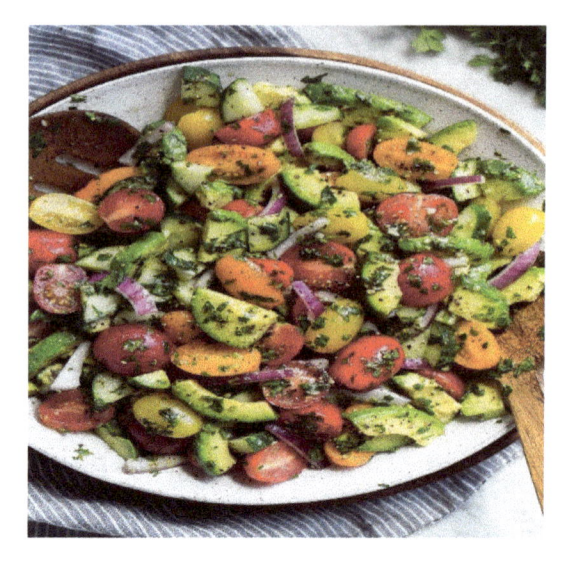

Berry Salad with Shrimps

Preparation Time: 7 minutes

Cooking Time: 0 minutes

Servings: 2

Ingredients:

- 1 cup corn kernels, cooked
- 1 endive, shredded
- 1 pound shrimp, cooked
- 1 tablespoon lime juice
- 2 cups raspberries, halved
- 2 tablespoons olive oil
- 1 tablespoon parsley, chopped

Directions:

1. Put all ingredients from the list above in the salad bowl and shake well.

Nutrition:

- 283 calories
- 29.5g protein
- 21.2g carbohydrates
- 10.1g fat
- 9.1g fiber
- 239mg cholesterol
- 313mg sodium

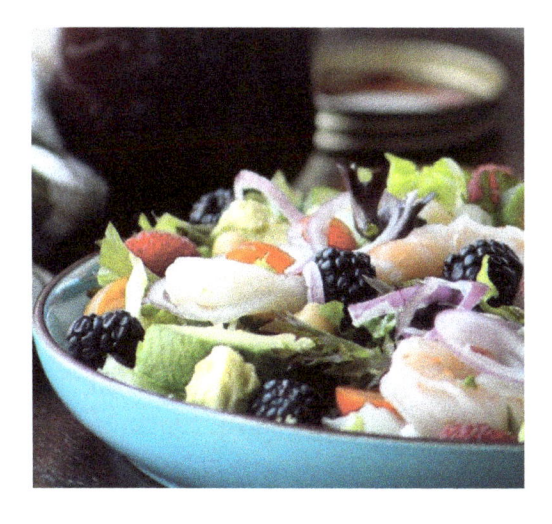

Sliced Mushrooms Salad

Preparation Time: 10 minutes

Cooking Time: 20 minutes

Servings: 2

Ingredients:

- 1 cup mushrooms, sliced
- 1 tablespoon margarine
- 1 cup lettuce, chopped
- 1 teaspoon lemon juice
- 1 tablespoon fresh dill, chopped
- 1 teaspoon cumin seeds

Directions:

2. Melt the margarine in the skillet.
3. Add mushrooms and lemon juice. Sauté the vegetables for 20 minutes over medium heat.
4. Then transfer the cooked mushrooms to the salad bowl, add lettuce, dill, and cumin seeds.
5. Stir the salad well.

Nutrition:

- 35 calories
- 0.9g protein
- 1.7g carbohydrates
- 3.1g fat
- 0.5g fiber
- 0mg cholesterol
- 38mg sodium

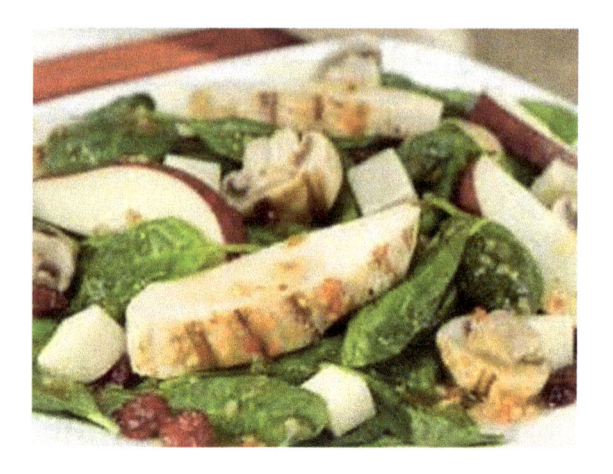

Tender Green Beans Salad

Preparation Time: 5 minutes

Cooking Time: 0 minutes

Servings: 2

Ingredients:

- 2 cups green beans, trimmed, chopped, cooked
- 2 tablespoons olive oil
- 2 pounds shrimp, cooked, peeled
- 1 cup tomato, chopped
- ¼ cup apple cider vinegar

Directions:

1. Mix up all ingredients together.
2. Then transfer the salad to the salad bowl.

Nutrition:

- 179 calories
- 26.5g protein
- 4.6g carbohydrates
- 5.5g fat
- 1.2g fiber
- 239mg cholesterol
- 280mg sodium

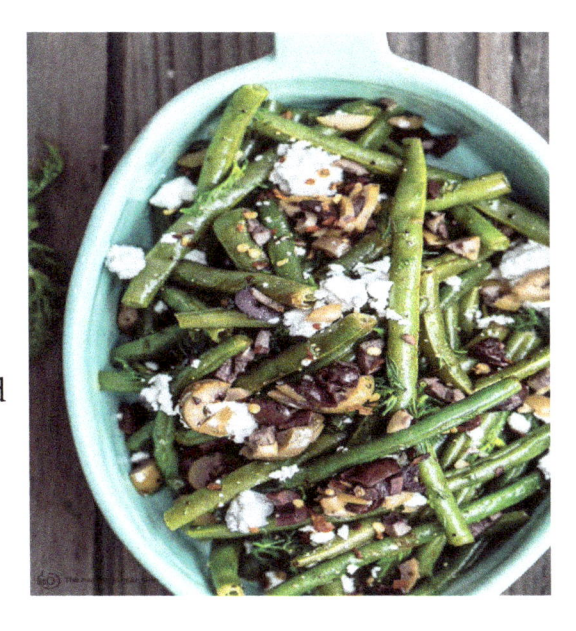

Spinach and Chicken Salad

Preparation Time: 7 minutes

Cooking Time: 0 minutes

Servings: 2

Ingredients:

- 1 tablespoon olive oil
- A pinch of black pepper
- 1-pound chicken breast, cooked, skinless, boneless, shredded
- 1 pound cherry tomatoes, halved
- 1 red onion, sliced
- 3 cups spinach, chopped
- 1 tablespoon lemon juice
- 1 tablespoon nuts, chopped

Directions:

1. Put all ingredients in the salad bowl and gently stir with the help of a spatula.

Nutrition:

- 209 calories
- 26.4g protein
- 8.4g carbohydrates
- 7.8g fat
- 2.7g fiber
- 73mg cholesterol
- 97mg sodium

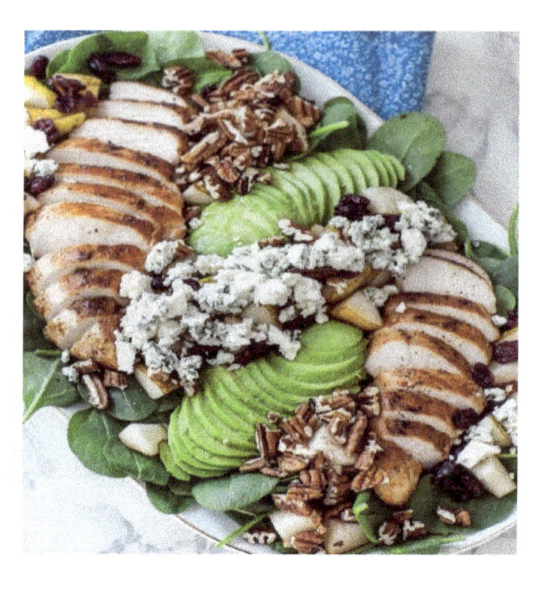

Cilantro Salad

Preparation Time: 10 minutes

Cooking Time: 8 minutes

Servings: 2

Ingredients:

- 1 tablespoon avocado oil
- 1 pound shrimp, peeled and deveined
- 2 cups lettuce, chopped
- 1 tablespoon balsamic vinegar
- 1 tablespoon lemon juice
- 1 cup fresh cilantro, chopped

Directions:

1. Heat up a pan with the oil over medium heat, add the shrimps and cook them for 4 minutes per side or until they are light brown.
2. Transfer the shrimps to the salad bowl and add all remaining ingredients from the list above. Shake the salad.

Nutrition:

- 146 calories
- 26.1g protein
- 3g carbohydrates
- 2.5g fat
- 0.5g fiber
- 239mg cholesterol
- 281mg sodium

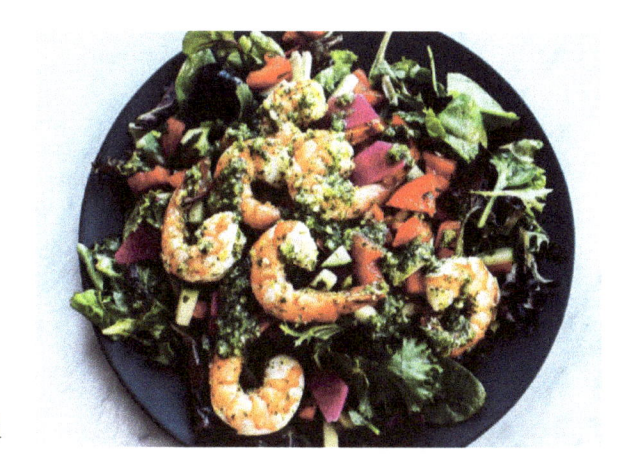

Iceberg Salad

Preparation Time: 10 minutes

Cooking Time: 0 minutes

Servings: 2

Ingredients:

- 1 cup iceberg lettuce, chopped
- 2 oz scallions, chopped
- 1 cup carrot, shredded
- 1 cup radish, sliced
- 2 tablespoons red vinegar
- ¼ cup olive oil

Directions:

1. Make the dressing: mix up olive oil and red vinegar.
2. Then mix up all remaining ingredients in the salad bowl.
3. Sprinkle the salad with dressing.

Nutrition:

- 130 calories
- 0.8g protein
- 5.1g carbohydrates
- 12.7g fat
- 1.6g fiber
- 0mg cholesterol
- 33mg sodium

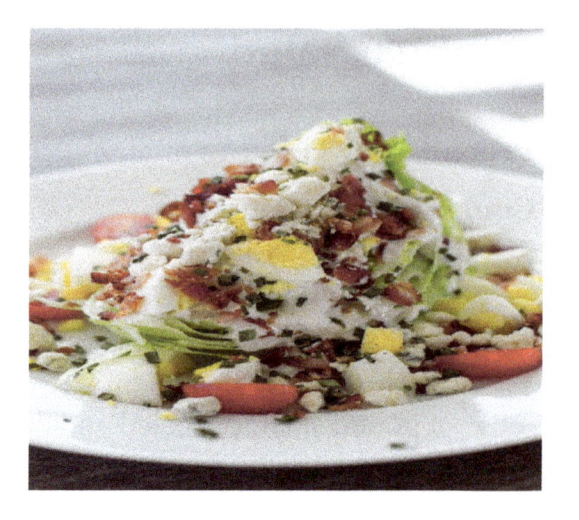

Seafood Salad with Grapes

Preparation Time: 5 minutes

Cooking Time: 0 minutes

Servings: 2

Ingredients:

- 2 tablespoons low-fat mayonnaise
- 2 teaspoons chili powder
- 1-pound shrimp, cooked, peeled
- 1 cup green grapes, halved
- 1 oz nuts, chopped

Directions:

1. Mix up all ingredients in the mixing bowl and transfer the salad to the serving plates.

Nutrition:

- 225 calories
- 27.4g protein
- 9.9g carbohydrates
- 8.3g fat
- 1.3g fiber
- 241mg cholesterol
- 390mg sodium

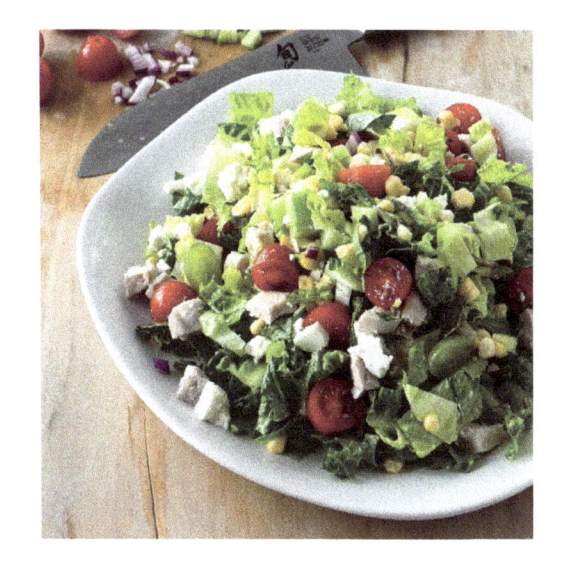

CHAPTER 4:

Soups & Stews

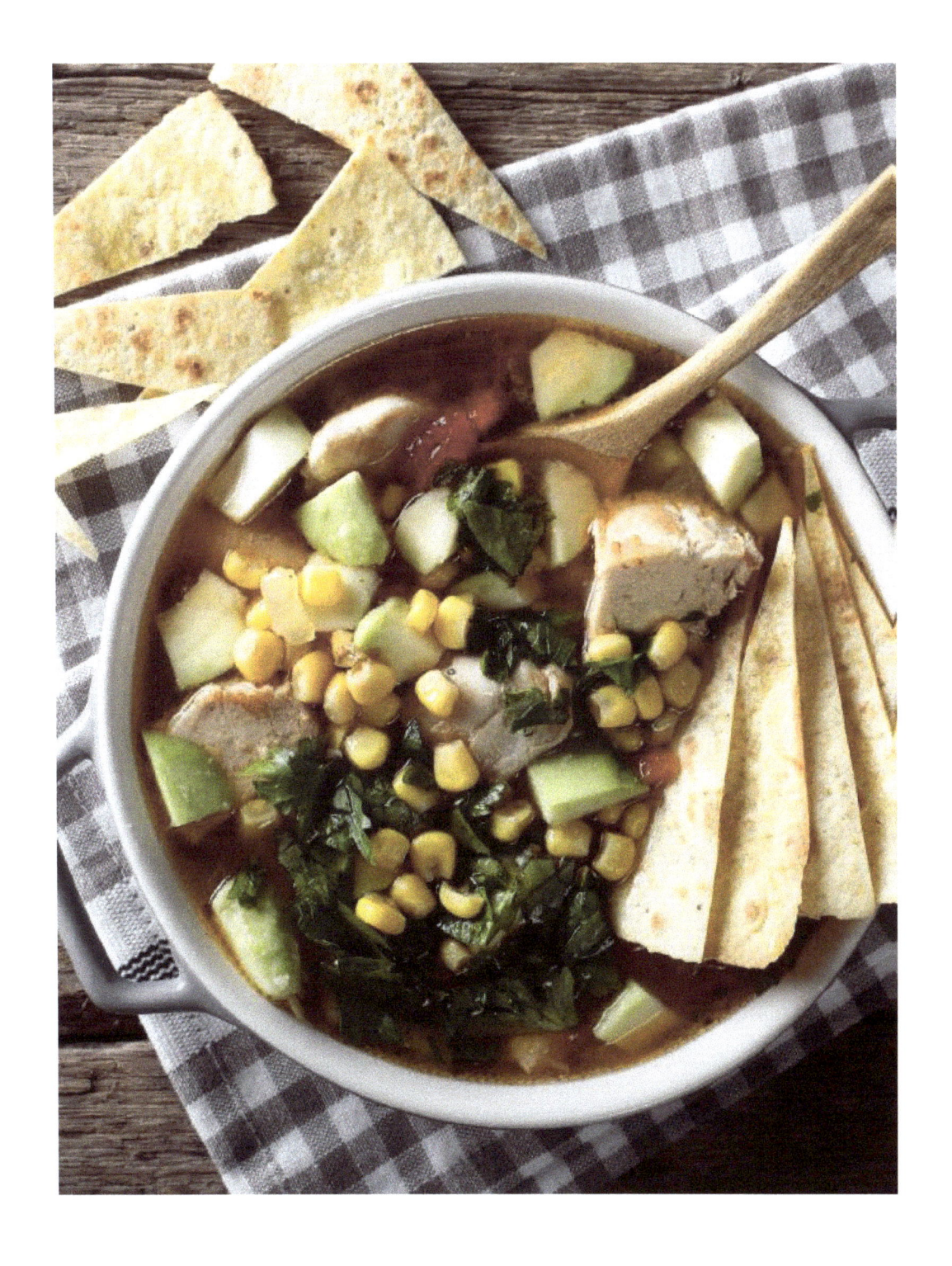

Pumpkin Cream Soup

Preparation Time: 10 minutes

Cooking Time: 20 minutes

Servings: 2

Ingredients:

- 1-pound pumpkin, chopped
- 1 teaspoon ground cumin
- ½ cup cauliflower, chopped
- 4 cups of water
- 1 teaspoon ground turmeric
- ½ teaspoon ground nutmeg
- 1 tablespoon fresh dill, chopped
- 1 teaspoon olive oil
- ½ cup skim milk

Directions:

1. Roast the pumpkin with olive oil in the saucepan for 3 minutes.
2. Then stir well and add cauliflower, cumin, turmeric, nutmeg, and water.
3. Close the lid and cook the soup on medium mode for 15 minutes or until the pumpkin is soft.
4. Then blend the mixture until smooth and add skim milk. Remove the soup from heat and top with dill.

Nutrition:

- 56 calories
- 2.2g protein
- 10g carbohydrates
- 1.4g fat
- 3.1g fiber
- 0mg cholesterol
- 28mg sodium

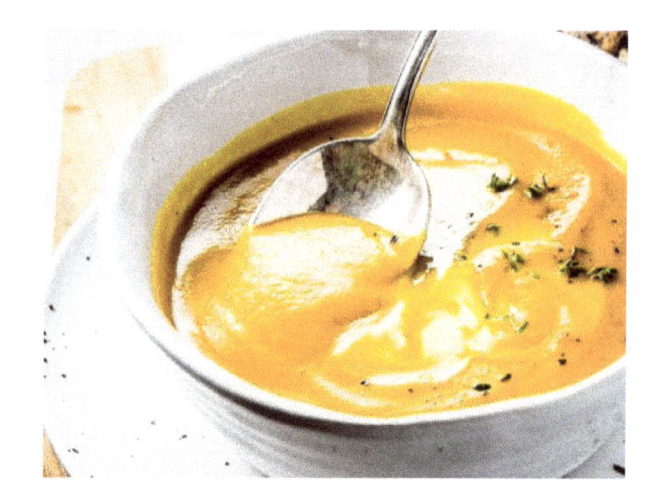

Zucchini Noodles Soup

Preparation Time: 10 minutes

Cooking Time: 15 minutes

Servings: 2

Ingredients:

- 2 zucchinis, trimmed
- 4 cups low-sodium chicken stock
- 2 oz fresh parsley, chopped
- ½ teaspoon chili flakes
- 1 oz carrot, shredded
- 1 teaspoon canola oil

Directions:

1. Roast the carrot with canola oil in the saucepan for 5 minutes over medium-low heat.
2. Stir it well and add chicken stock. Bring the mixture to a boil.
3. Meanwhile, make the noodles from the zucchini with the help of the spiralizer.
4. Add them to the boiling soup liquid.
5. Add parsley and chili flakes. Bring the soup to a boil and remove it from the heat.
6. Leave for 10 minutes to rest.

Nutrition:

- 39 calories
- 2.7g protein
- 4.9g carbohydrates
- 1.5g fat
- 1.7g fiber
- 0mg cholesterol
- 158mg sodium

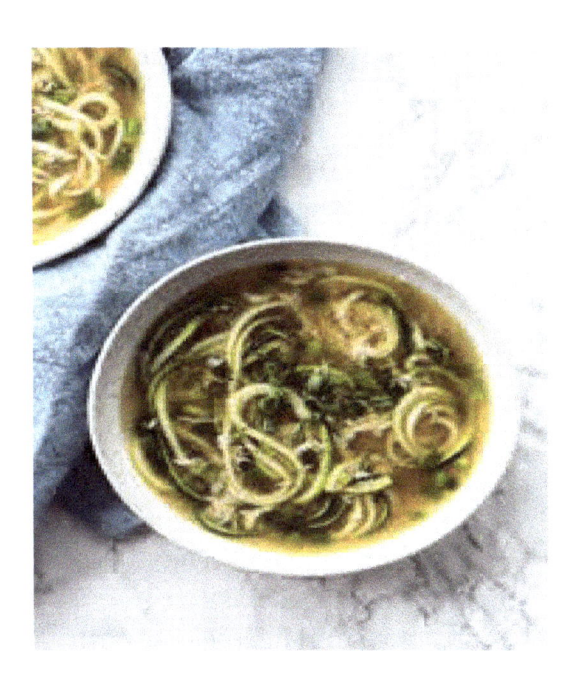

Grilled Tomatoes Soup

Preparation Time: 10 minutes

Cooking Time: 20 minutes

Servings: 1

Ingredients:

- 2-pounds tomatoes
- ½ cup shallot, chopped
- 1 tablespoon avocado oil
- ½ teaspoon ground black pepper
- ¼ teaspoon minced garlic
- 1 tablespoon dried basil
- 3 cups low-sodium chicken broth

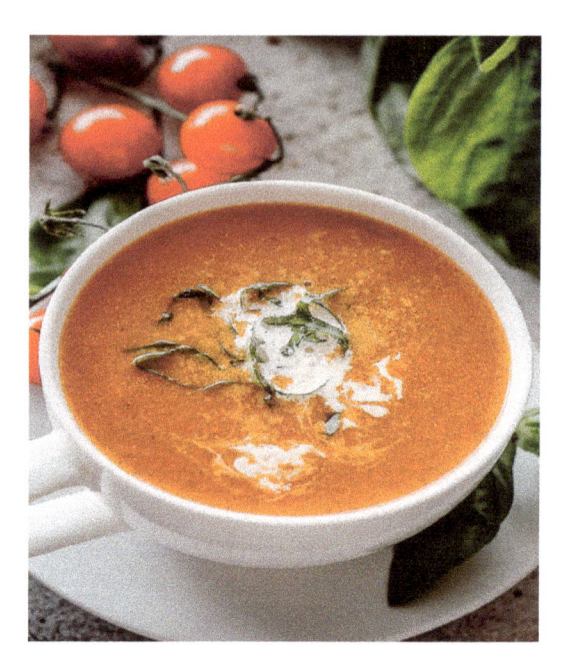

Directions:

1. Cut the tomatoes into halves and grill them in the preheated to 390F grill for 1 minute from each side.
2. After this, transfer the grilled tomatoes to the blender and blend until smooth.
3. Place the shallot and avocado oil in the saucepan and roast it until light brown.
4. Add blended grilled tomatoes, ground black pepper, and minced garlic.
5. Bring the soup to a boil and sprinkle with dried basil.
6. Simmer the soup for 2 minutes more.

Nutrition:

- 72 calories
- 4.1g protein
- 13.4g carbohydrates
- 0.9g fat
- 3g fiber
- 0mg cholesterol
- 98mg sodium

Chicken Oatmeal Soup

Preparation Time: 10 minutes

Cooking Time: 15 minutes

Servings: 2

Ingredients:

- 1 cup oats
- 4 cups of water
- 1 oz fresh dill, chopped
- 10 oz chicken fillet, chopped
- 1 teaspoon ground black pepper
- 1 teaspoon potato starch
- ½ carrot, diced

Directions:

1. Put the chopped chicken in the saucepan, add water, and bring it to a boil. Simmer the chicken for 10 minutes.
2. Add dill, ground black pepper, oats, and diced carrot.
3. Bring the soup to a boil and add potato starch. Stir it until the soup starts to thicken. Simmer the soup for 5 minutes on low heat.

Nutrition:

- 192 calories
- 19.8g protein
- 16.1g carbohydrates
- 5.5g fat
- 2.7g fiber
- 50mg cholesterol
- 72mg sodium

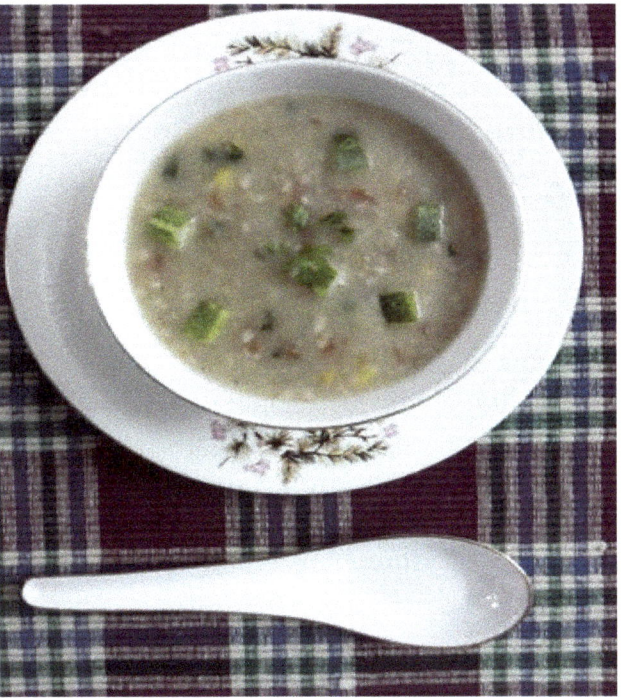

Celery Cream Soup

Preparation Time: 10 minutes

Cooking Time: 25 minutes

Servings: 1

Ingredients:

- 2 cups celery stalk, chopped
- 1 shallot, chopped
- 1 potato, chopped
- 4 cups low-sodium vegetable stock
- 1 tablespoon margarine
- 1 teaspoon white pepper

Directions:

1. Melt the margarine in the saucepan, add shallot, and celery stalk. Cook the vegetables for 5 minutes. Stir them occasionally.
2. After this, add vegetable stock and potato.
3. Simmer the soup for 15 minutes.
4. Blend the soup until you get the creamy texture and sprinkle with white pepper.
5. Simmer it for 5 minutes more.

Nutrition:

- 88 calories
- 2.3g protein
- 13.3g carbohydrates
- 3g fat
- 2.9g fiber
- 0mg cholesterol
- 217mg sodium
- 449mg potassium

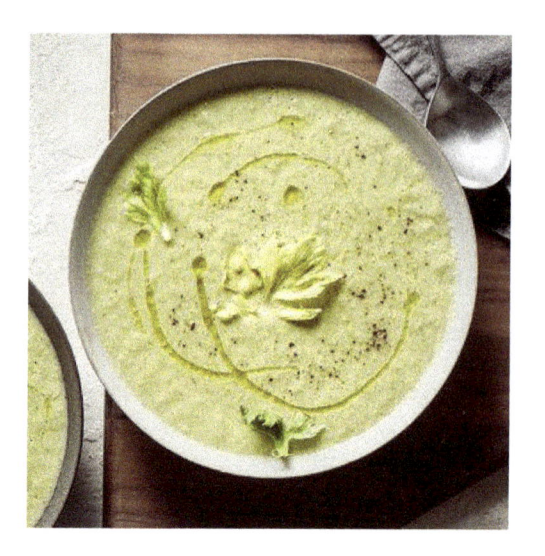

Cauliflower Soup

Preparation Time: 10 minutes

Cooking Time: 20 minutes

Servings: 2

Ingredients:

- 1 cup cauliflower, chopped
- ¼ cup potato, chopped
- 1 cup skim milk
- 1 cup of water
- 1 teaspoon ground coriander
- 1 teaspoon margarine

Directions:

1. Put cauliflower and potato in the saucepan.
2. Add water and boil the ingredients for 15 minutes.
3. Then add ground coriander and margarine.
4. With the help of the immersion blender, blend the soup until smooth.
5. Add skim milk and stir well.

Nutrition:

- 82 calories
- 5.2g protein
- 10.3g carbohydrates
- 2g fat
- 1.5g fiber
- 2mg cholesterol
- 106mg sodium

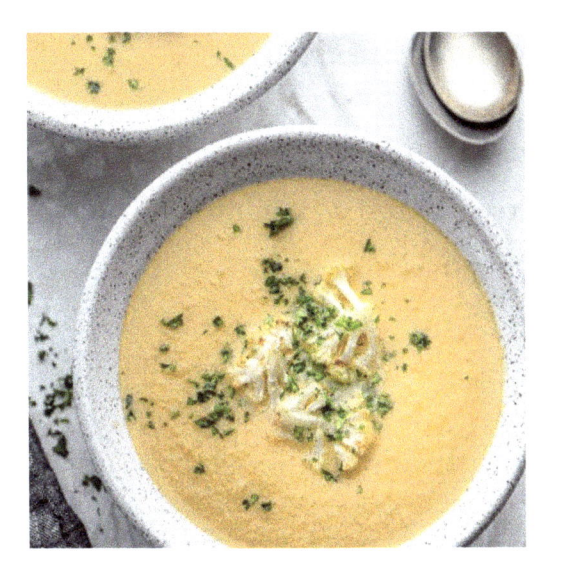

Buckwheat Soup

Preparation Time: 10 minutes

Cooking Time: 25 minutes

Servings: 2

Ingredients:

- ½ cup buckwheat
- 1 carrot, chopped
- 1 yellow onion, diced
- 1 tablespoon avocado oil
- 1 tablespoon fresh dill, chopped
- 1-pound chicken breast, chopped
- 1 teaspoon ground black pepper
- 6 cups of water

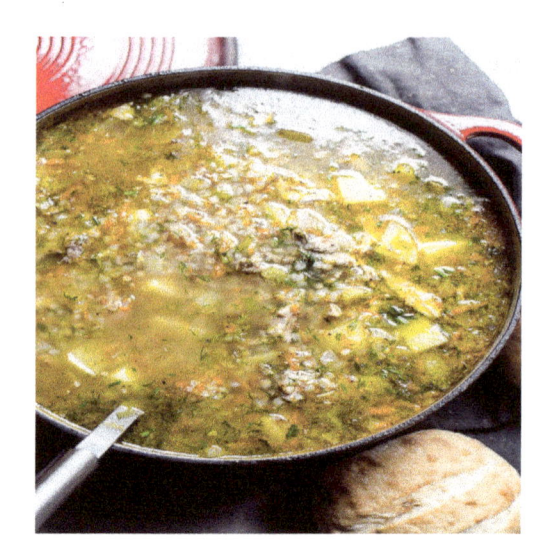

Directions:

1. Sauté the onion, carrot, and avocado oil in the saucepan for 5 minutes. Stir them from time to time.
2. Then add buckwheat, chicken breast, and ground black pepper.
3. Add water and close the lid.
4. Simmer the soup for 20 minutes.
5. After this, add dill and remove the soup from the heat. Leave it for 10 minutes to rest.

Nutrition:

- 152 calories
- 18.4g protein
- 13.5g carbohydrates
- 2.7g fat
- 2.3g fiber
- 48mg cholesterol
- 48mg sodium

Parsley Soup

Preparation Time: 10 minutes

Cooking Time: 16 minutes

Servings: 2

Ingredients:

- 2 teaspoons olive oil
- 1 cup carrot, shredded
- 1 cup yellow onion, chopped
- 1 cup celery, chopped
- 6 cups of water
- 1 cup fresh parsley, chopped
- ¼ cup low-fat parmesan, grated

Directions:

1. Heat up a pot with the oil over medium-high heat, add onion, carrot, and celery, stir and cook for 7 minutes.
2. Add water and all remaining ingredients.
3. Cook the soup for 8 minutes over medium heat.

Nutrition:

- 46 calories
- 1.6g protein
- 4.8g carbohydrates
- 2.5g fat
- 1.5g fiber
- 4mg cholesterol
- 103mg sodium

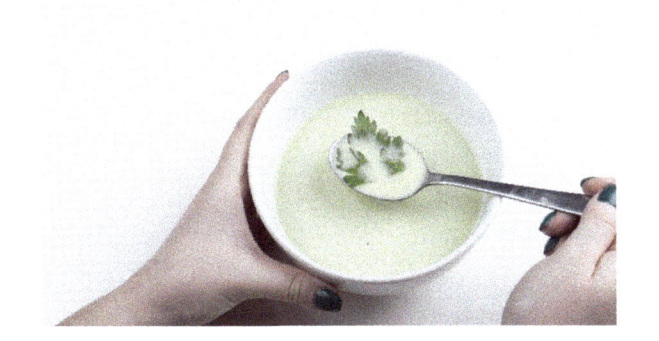

Tomato Bean Soup

Preparation Time: 10 minutes

Cooking Time: 25 minutes

Servings: 1

Ingredients:

- 2 teaspoons olive oil
- 2 garlic cloves, minced
- 1 pound green beans, trimmed and halved
- 4 tomatoes, cubed
- 1 teaspoon sweet paprika
- 4 cup of water
- 2 tablespoons dill, chopped

Directions:

1. Heat up a pot with the oil over medium-high heat, add the garlic stir. Sauté the garlic for 5 minutes.
2. Add all remaining ingredients and cook the soup for 20 minutes.

Nutrition:

- 57 calories
- 2.4g protein
- 9.7g carbohydrates
- 1.9g fat
- 3.8g fiber
- 0mg cholesterol
- 16mg sodium

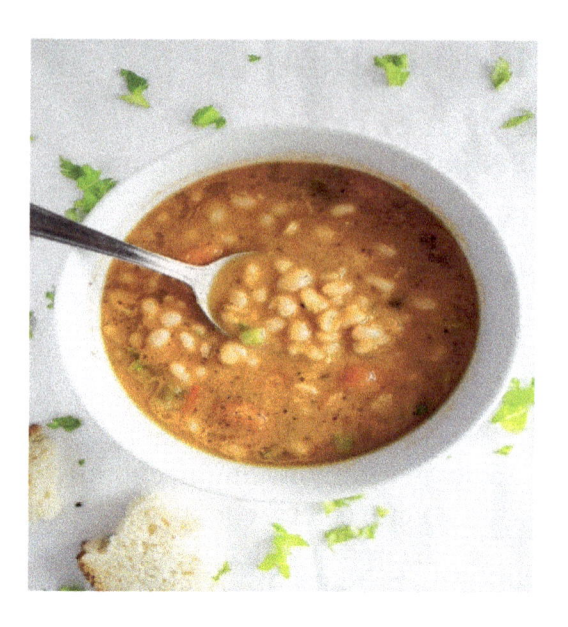

Red Kidney Beans Soup

Preparation Time: 10 minutes

Cooking Time: 20 minutes

Servings: 2

Ingredients:

- 2 teaspoons olive oil
- 1 yellow onion, chopped
- 1 teaspoon cinnamon powder
- 1 cup red kidney beans, cooked
- 3 cups low-sodium chicken broth
- 1 potato, chopped

Directions:

1. Heat up a pot with the oil over medium heat, add onion and cinnamon, stir and cook for 6 minutes.
2. Add all remaining ingredients and cook them for 14 minutes.
3. Blend the soup until you get a puree texture.

Nutrition:

- 230 calories
- 13g protein
- 38.9g carbohydrates
- 2.9g fat
- 8.5g fiber
- 0mg cholesterol
- 62mg sodium

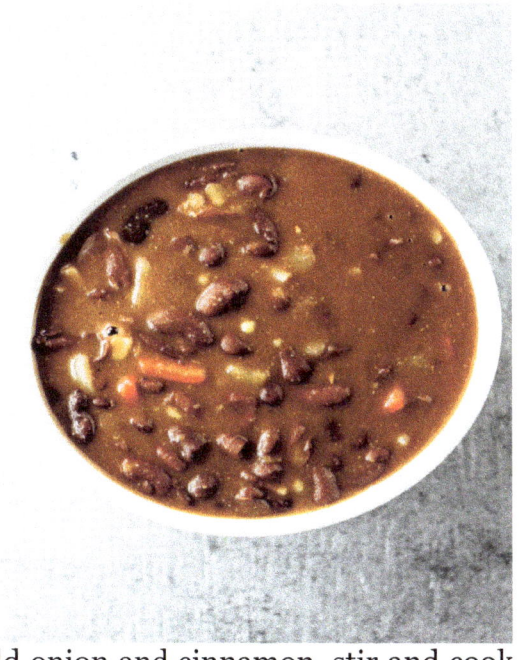

Pork Soup

Preparation Time: 10 minutes

Cooking Time: 25 minutes

Servings: 2

Ingredients:

- 1 tablespoon avocado oil
- 1 onion, chopped
- 1 pound pork stew meat, cubed
- 4 cups of water
- 1 pound carrots, sliced
- 1 teaspoon tomato paste

Directions:

1. Heat up a pot with the oil over medium-high heat, add the onion and pork, and cook the ingredients for 5 minutes.
2. Add all remaining ingredients and cook the soup for 20 minutes.

Nutrition:

- 304 calories
- 34.5g protein
- 14.2g carbohydrates
- 11.4g fat
- 3.6g fiber
- 98mg cholesterol
- 155mg sodium

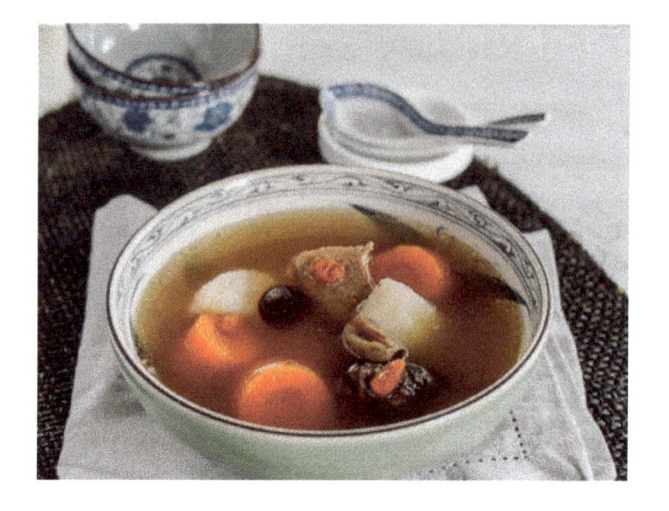

Curry Soup

Preparation Time: 10 minutes

Cooking Time: 23 minutes

Servings: 2

Ingredients:

- 3 tablespoons olive oil
- 8 carrots, peeled and sliced
- 2 teaspoons curry paste
- 4 celery stalks, chopped
- 1 yellow onion, chopped
- 4 cups of water

Directions:

1. Heat up a pot with the oil and add onion, celery and carrots, stir and cook for 12 minutes.
2. Then add curry paste and water. Stir the soup well and cook it for 10 minutes more.
3. When all ingredients are soft, blend the soup until smooth and simmer it for 1 minute more.

Nutrition:

- 171 calories
- 1.6g protein
- 15.8g carbohydrates
- 12g fat
- 3.9g fiber
- 0mg cholesterol
- 106mg sodium

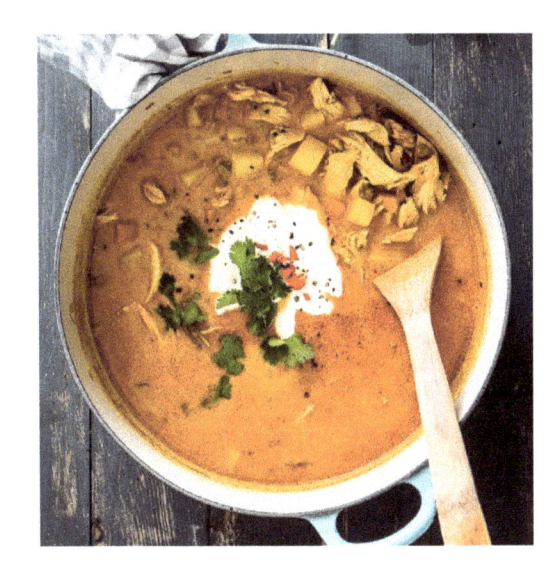

Yellow Onion Soup

Preparation Time: 10 minutes

Cooking Time: 20 minutes

Servings: 2

Ingredients:

- 1 tablespoon avocado oil
- 1 yellow onion, chopped
- 1 teaspoon ginger, grated
- 1 pound zucchinis, chopped
- 4 cups low-sodium chicken broth
- ½ cup low-fat cream
- 1 teaspoon ground black pepper

Directions:

1. Heat up a pot with the oil over medium heat, add the onion and ginger, stir and cook for 5 minutes.
2. Add all remaining ingredients and simmer them over medium heat for 15 minutes.
3. Blend the cooked soup and ladle in the bowls.

Nutrition:

- 61 calories
- 4.2g protein
- 10.2g carbohydrates
- 0.7g fat
- 2.2g fiber
- 1mg cholesterol
- 101mg sodium

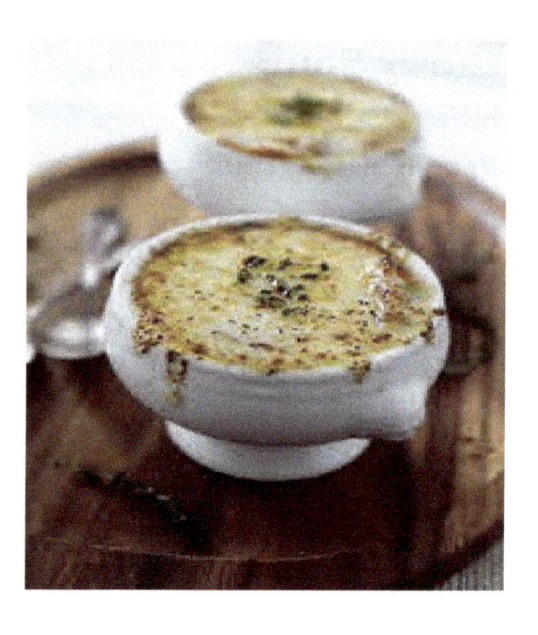

Garlic Soup

Preparation Time: 10 minutes

Cooking Time: 50 minutes

Servings: 2

Ingredients:

- 1 pound red kidney beans, cooked
- 8 cups of water
- 1 green bell pepper, chopped
- 1 tomato paste
- 1 yellow onion, chopped
- 1 teaspoon minced garlic
- 1 pound beef sirloin, cubed
- 1 teaspoon garlic powder

Directions:

1. Pour water into a pot and heat up over medium heat.
2. Add all ingredients and close the lid.
3. Simmer the soup for 45 minutes over medium heat.

Nutrition:

- 620 calories
- 60.9g protein
- 75.8g carbohydrates
- 8.4g fat
- 18.5g fiber
- 101mg cholesterol
- 109mg sodium

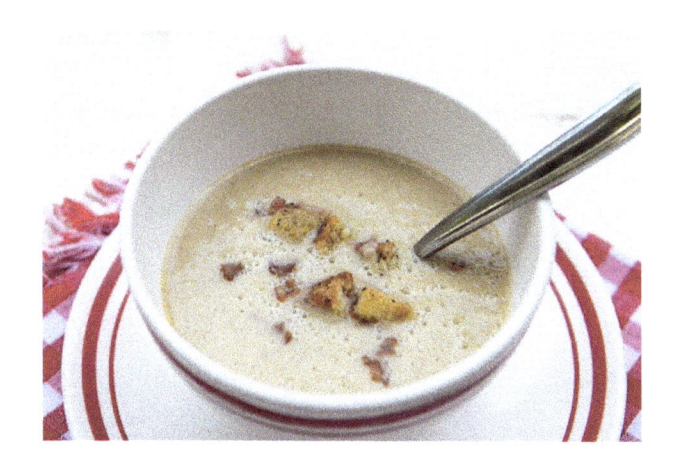

CHAPTER 5:

Vegan & Vegetarian

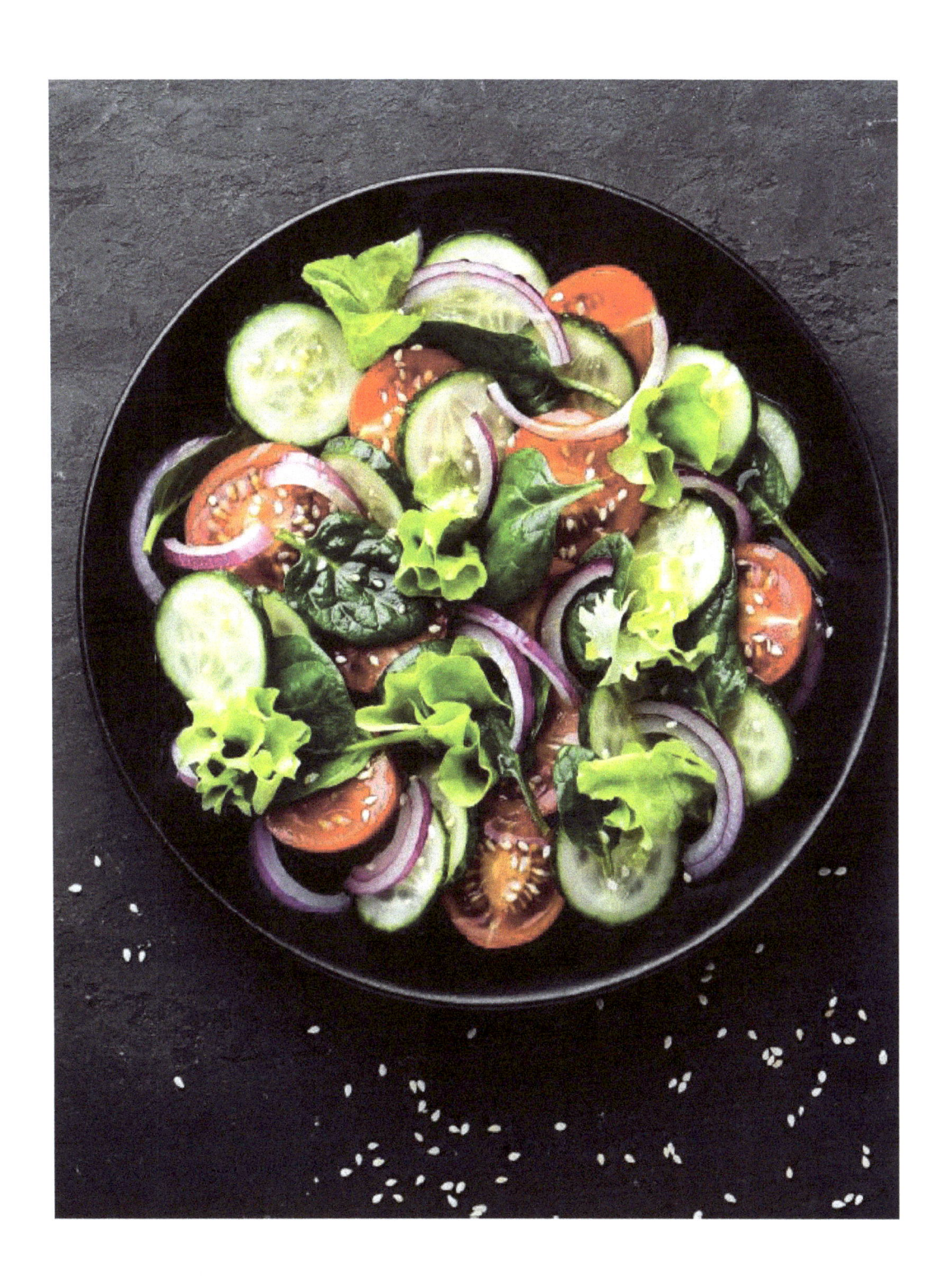

Chickpea Curry

Preparation Time: 10 minutes

Cooking Time: 10 minutes

Servings: 2

Ingredients:

- 1 ½ cup chickpeas, boiled
- 1 teaspoon curry powder
- ½ teaspoon garam masala
- 1 cup spinach, chopped
- 1 teaspoon coconut oil
- ¼ cup of soy milk
- 1 tablespoon tomato paste
- ½ cup of water

Directions:

1. Heat up coconut oil in the saucepan.
2. Add curry powder, garam masala, tomato paste, and soy milk.
3. Whisk the mixture until smooth and bring it to a boil.
4. Add water, spinach, and chickpeas.
5. Stir the meal and close the lid.
6. Cook it for 5 minutes over medium heat.

Nutrition:

- 298 calories
- 15.4g protein
- 47.8g carbohydrates
- 6.1g fat
- 13.6g fiber
- 0mg cholesterol
- 37mg sodium

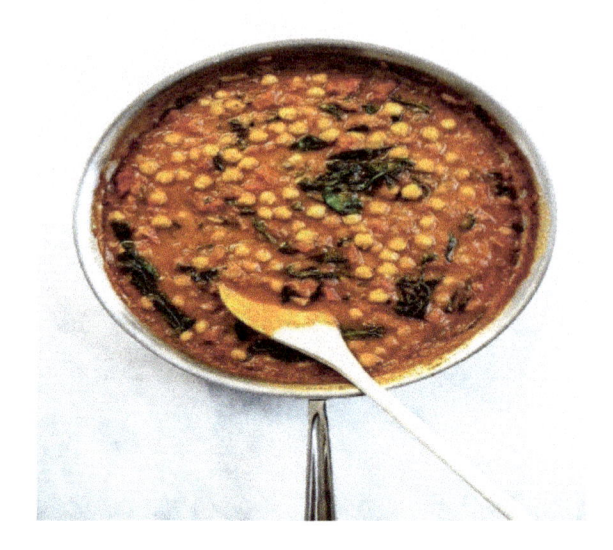

Quinoa Bowl

Preparation Time: 15 minutes

Cooking Time: 15 minutes

Servings: 1

Ingredients:

- 1 cup quinoa
- 2 cups of water
- 1 cup tomatoes, diced
- 1 cup sweet pepper, diced
- ½ cup of rice, cooked
- 1 tablespoon lemon juice
- ½ teaspoon lemon zest, grated
- 1 tablespoon olive oil

Directions:

1. Mix up water and quinoa and cook it for 15 minutes. Then remove it from the heat and leave to rest for 10 minutes.
2. Transfer the cooked quinoa to the big bowl.
3. Add tomatoes, sweet pepper, rice, lemon juice, lemon zest, and olive oil.
4. Stir the mixture well and transfer to the serving bowls.

Nutrition:

- 290 calories
- 8.4g protein
- 49.9g carbohydrates
- 6.4g fat
- 4.3g fiber
- 0mg cholesterol
- 11mg sodium

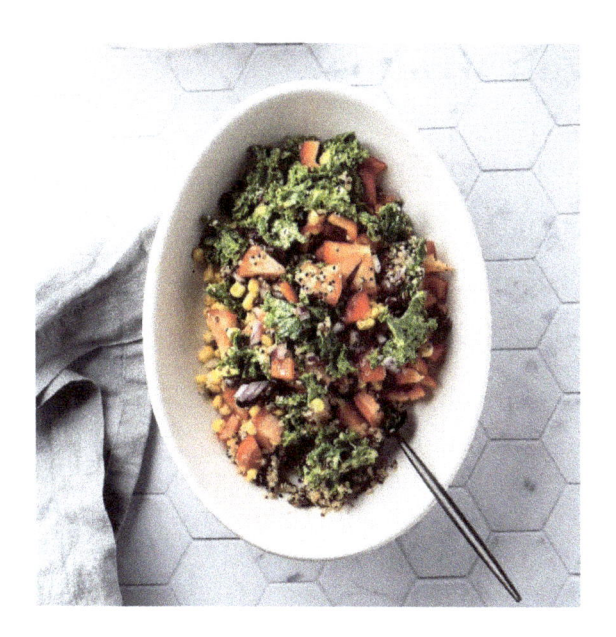

Vegan Meatloaf

Preparation Time: 10 minutes

Cooking Time: 30 minutes

Servings: 2

Ingredients:

- 1 cup chickpeas, cooked
- 1 onion, diced
- 1 tablespoon ground flax seeds
- ½ teaspoon chili flakes
- 1 tablespoon coconut oil
- ½ cup carrot, diced
- ½ cup celery stalk, chopped
- 1 tablespoon tomato paste

Directions:

1. Heat up coconut oil in the saucepan.
2. Add carrot, onion, and celery stalk. Cook the vegetables for 8 minutes or until they are soft.
3. Then add chickpeas, chili flakes, and ground flax seeds.
4. Blend the mixture until smooth with the help of the immersion blender.
5. Then line the loaf mold with baking paper and transfer the blended mixture inside.
6. Flatten it well and spread with tomato paste.
7. Bake the meatloaf in the preheated to 365F oven for 20 minutes.

Nutrition:

- 162 calories
- 7.1g protein
- 23.9g carbohydrates
- 4.7g fat
- 7g fiber
- 0mg cholesterol
- 25mg sodium

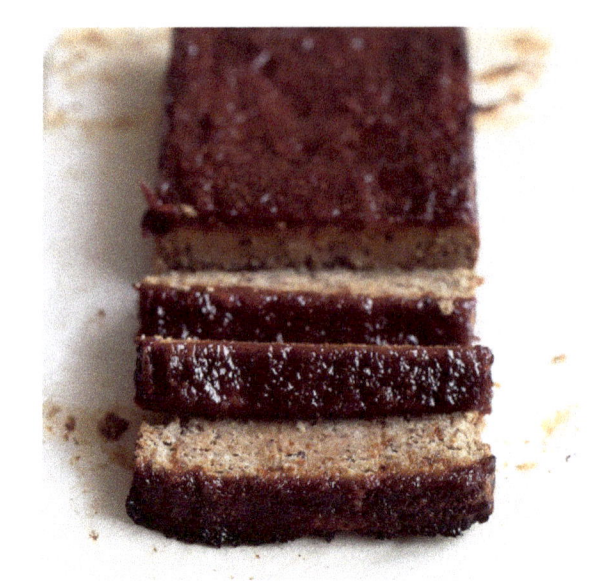

Loaded Potato Skins

Preparation Time: 15 minutes

Cooking Time: 45 minutes

Servings: 2

Ingredients:

- 6 potatoes
- 1 teaspoon ground black pepper
- 2 tablespoons olive oil
- ½ teaspoon minced garlic
- ¼ cup of soy milk

Directions:

1. Preheat the oven to 400F.
2. Pierce the potatoes with the help of the knife 2-3 times and bake in the oven for 30 minutes or until the vegetables are tender.
3. After this, cut the baked potatoes into halves and scoop out the potato meat in the bowl.
4. Sprinkle the scooped potato halves with olive oil and ground black pepper and return them back to the oven. Bake them for 15 minutes or until they are light brown.
5. Meanwhile, mash the scooped potato meat and mix it up with soy milk and minced garlic.
6. Fill the cooked potato halves with the mashed potato mixture.

Nutrition:

- 194 calories
- 4g protein
- 34.4g carbohydrates
- 5.1g fat
- 5.3g fiber
- 0mg cholesterol
- 18mg sodium

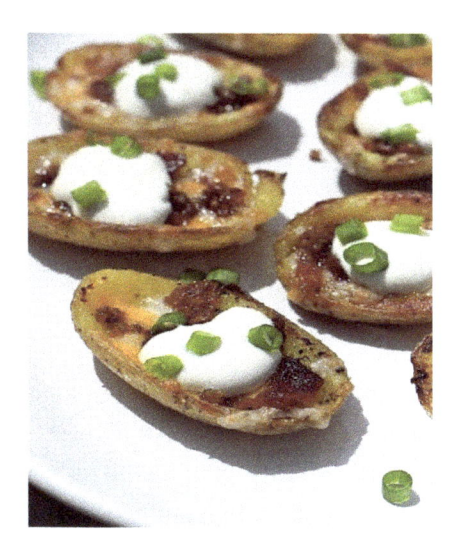

Vegan Shepherd Pie

Preparation Time: 15 minutes

Cooking Time: 35 minutes

Servings: 2

Ingredients:

- ½ cup quinoa, cooked
- ½ cup tomato puree
- ½ cup carrot, diced
- 1 shallot, chopped
- 1 tablespoon coconut oil
- ½ cup potato, cooked, mashed
- 1 teaspoon chili powder
- ½ cup mushrooms, sliced

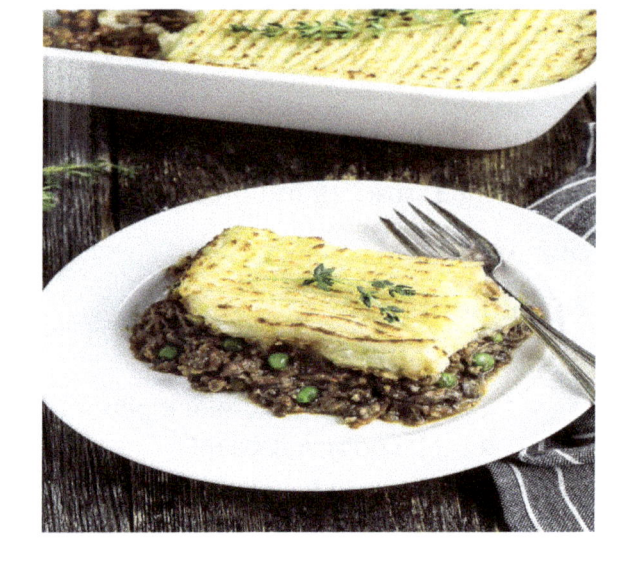

Directions:

1. Put carrot, shallot, and mushrooms in the saucepan.
2. Add coconut oil and cook the vegetables for 10 minutes or until they are tender but not soft.
3. Then mix up cooked vegetables with chili powder and tomato puree.
4. Transfer the mixture to the casserole mold and flatten well.
5. After this, top the vegetables with mashed potatoes. Cover the shepherd pie with foil and bake in the preheated to 375F oven for 25 minutes.

Nutrition:

- 136 calories
- 4.2g protein
- 20.1g carbohydrates
- 4.9g fat
- 2.9g fiber
- 0mg cholesterol
- 27mg sodium

Cauliflower Steaks

Preparation Time: 15 minutes

Cooking Time: 25 minutes

Servings: 2

Ingredients:

- 1-pound cauliflower head
- 1 teaspoon ground turmeric
- ½ teaspoon cayenne pepper
- 2 tablespoons olive oil
- ½ teaspoon garlic powder

Directions:

1. Slice the cauliflower head into the steaks and rub with ground turmeric, cayenne pepper, and garlic powder.
2. Then line the baking tray with baking paper and put the cauliflower steaks inside.
3. Sprinkle them with olive oil and bake at 375F for 25 minutes or until the vegetable steaks are tender.

Nutrition:

- 92 calories
- 2.4g protein
- 6.8g carbohydrates
- 7.2g fat
- 3.1g fiber
- 0mg cholesterol
- 34mg sodium

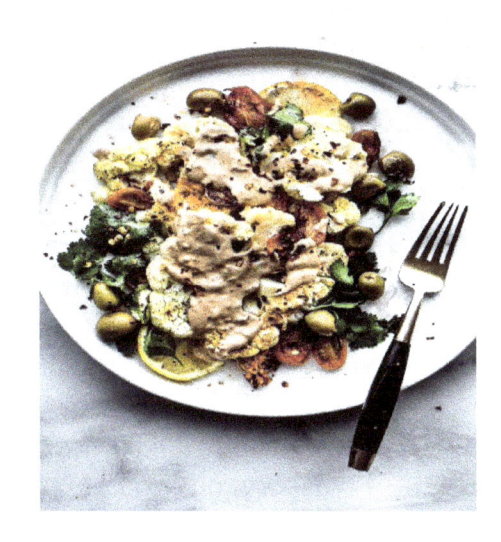

Quinoa Burger

Preparation Time: 15 minutes

Cooking Time: 20 minutes

Servings: 2

Ingredients:

- 1/3 cup chickpeas, cooked
- ½ cup quinoa, cooked
- 1 teaspoon Italian seasonings
- 1 teaspoon olive oil
- ½ onion, minced

Directions:

1. Blend the chickpeas until they are smooth.
2. Then mix them up with quinoa, Italian seasonings, and minced onion. Stir the ingredients until homogenous.
3. After this, make the burgers from the mixture and place them in the lined baking tray.
4. Sprinkle the quinoa burgers with olive oil and bake them at 275F for 20 minutes.

Nutrition:

- 158 calories
- 6.4g protein
- 25.2g carbohydrates
- 3.8g fat
- 4.7g fiber
- 1mg cholesterol
- 6mg sodium

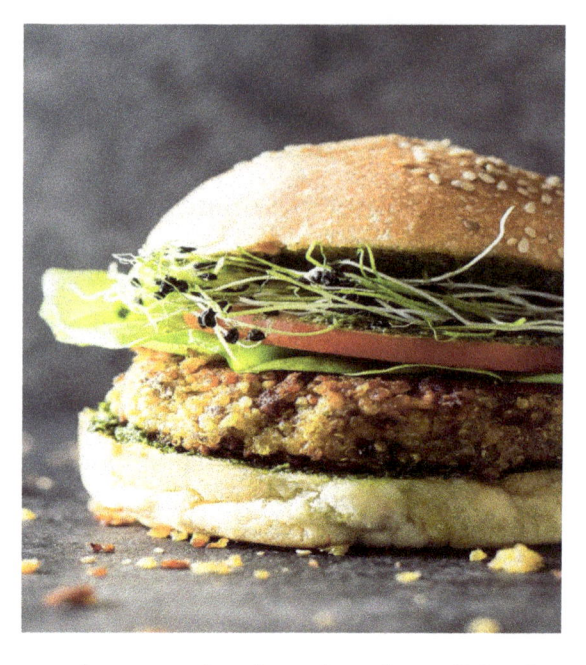

Cauliflower Tots

Preparation Time: 15 minutes

Cooking Time: 20 minutes

Servings: 1

Ingredients:

- 1 cup cauliflower, shredded
- 3 oz vegan Parmesan, grated
- 1/3 cup flax seeds meal
- 1 egg, beaten
- 1 teaspoon Italian seasonings
- 1 teaspoon olive oil

Directions:

1. In the bowl mix up shredded cauliflower, vegan Parmesan, flax seeds meal, egg, and Italian seasonings.
2. Knead the cauliflower mixture. Add water if needed.
3. After this, make the cauliflower tots from the mixture.
4. Line the baking tray with baking paper and place the cauliflower tots inside.
5. Sprinkle them with the olive oil and transfer in the preheated to 375F oven.
6. Bake the meal for 15-20 minutes or until golden brown.

Nutrition:

- 109 calories
- 6.1g protein
- 6.3g carbohydrates
- 6.6g fat
- 3.7g fiber
- 42mg cholesterol
- 72mg sodium

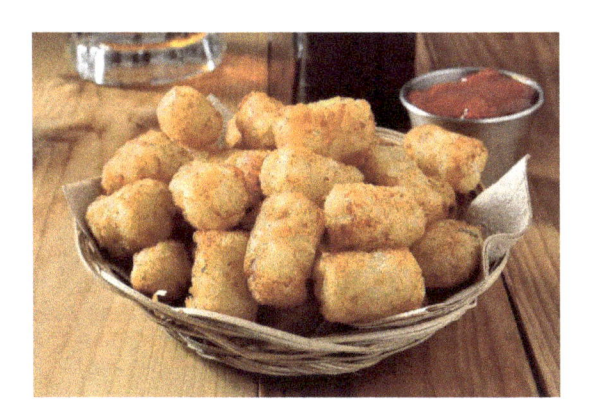

Zucchini Soufflé

Preparation Time: 10 minutes

Cooking Time: 60 minutes

Servings: 2

Ingredients:

- 2 cups zucchini, grated
- ½ teaspoon baking powder
- ½ cup oatmeal, grinded
- 1 onion, diced
- 3 tablespoons water
- 1 teaspoon cayenne pepper
- 1 teaspoon dried thyme

Directions:

1. Mix up all ingredients together in the casserole mold.
2. Flatten well the zucchini mixture and cover with foil.
3. Bake the soufflé at 365F for 60 minutes.

Nutrition:

- 41 calories
- 1.6g protein
- 8.1g carbohydrates
- 0.6g fat
- 1.6g fiber
- 0mg cholesterol
- 6mg sodium

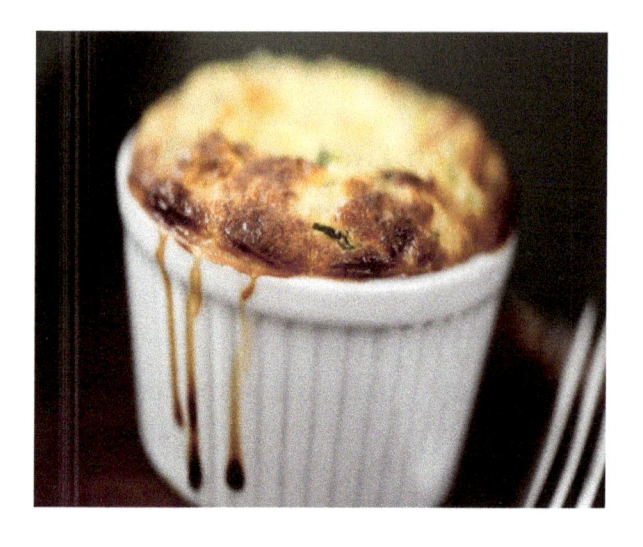

Honey Sweet Potato Bake

Preparation Time: 20 minutes

Cooking Time: 20 minutes

Servings: 2

Ingredients:

- 4 sweet potatoes, baked
- 1 tablespoon honey
- 1 teaspoon ground cinnamon
- ¼ teaspoon ground cardamom
- 1/3 cup soy milk

Directions:

1. Peel the sweet potatoes and mash them.
2. Then mix mashed potato with ground cinnamon, cardamom, and soy milk. Stir it well.
3. Transfer the mixture to the baking pan and flatten well.
4. Sprinkle the mixture with honey and cover with foil.
5. Bake the meal at 375F for 20 minutes.

Nutrition:

- 30 calories
- 0.7g protein
- 6.5g carbohydrates
- 0.4g fat
- 0.5g fiber
- 0mg cholesterol
- 11mg sodium

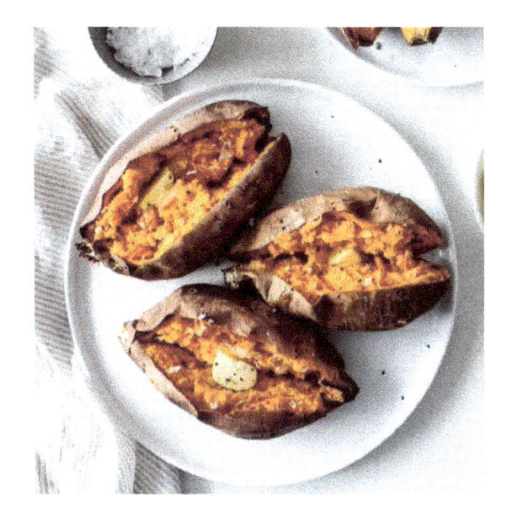

Lentil Quiche

Preparation Time: 15 minutes

Cooking Time: 35 minutes

Servings: 2

Ingredients:

- 1 cup green lentils, boiled
- ½ cup carrot, grated
- 1 onion, diced
- 1 tablespoon olive oil
- ¼ cup flax seeds meal
- 1 teaspoon ground black pepper
- ¼ cup of soy milk

Directions:

1. Cook the onion with olive oil in the skillet until light brown.
2. Then mix up cooked onion, lentils, and carrot.
3. Add flax seeds meal, ground black pepper, and soy milk. Stir the mixture until homogenous.
4. After this, transfer it to the baking pan and flatten it.
5. Bake the quiche for 35 minutes at 375F.

Nutrition:

- 351 calories
- 17.1g protein
- 41.6g carbohydrates
- 13.1g fat
- 23.3g fiber
- 0mg cholesterol
- 29mg sodium

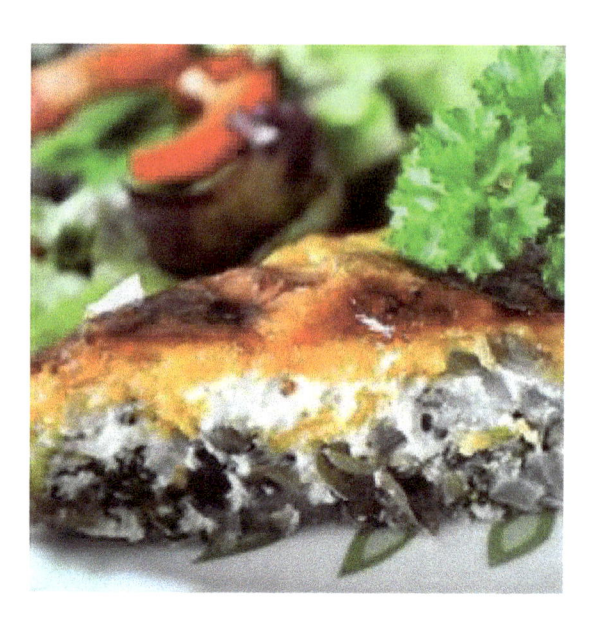

Corn Patties

Preparation Time: 15 minutes

Cooking Time: 10 minutes

Servings: 1

Ingredients:

- ½ cup chickpeas, cooked
- 1 cup corn kernels, cooked
- 1 tablespoon fresh parsley, chopped
- 1 teaspoon chili powder
- ½ teaspoon ground coriander
- 1 tablespoon tomato paste
- 1 tablespoon almond meal
- 1 tablespoon olive oil

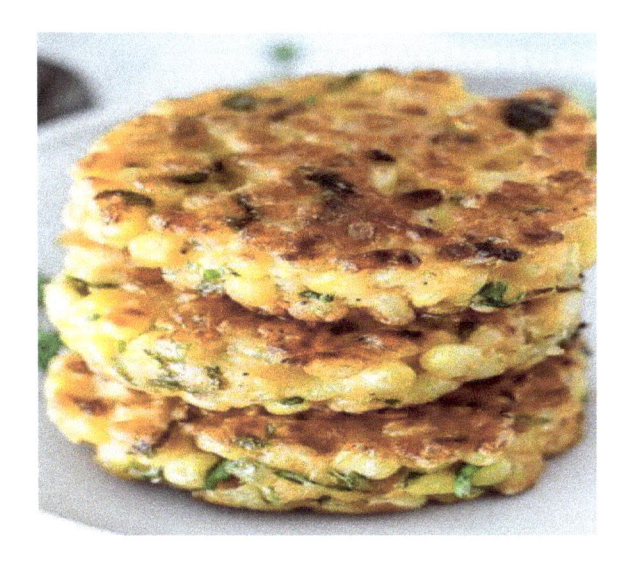

Directions:

1. Mash the cooked chickpeas and combine them with corn kernels, parsley, chili powder, ground coriander, tomato paste, and almond meal.
2. Stir the mixture until homogenous.
3. Make the small patties.
4. After this, heat up olive oil in the skillet.
5. Put the prepared patties in the hot oil and cook them for 3 minutes per side or until they are golden brown.
6. Dry the cooked patties with the help of paper towel if needed.

Nutrition:

- 168 calories
- 6.7g protein
- 23.9g carbohydrates
- 6.3g fat,
- 6g fiber
- 0mg cholesterol
- 23mg sodium

Tofu Stir Fry

Preparation Time: 15 minutes

Cooking Time: 10 minutes

Servings: 2

Ingredients:

- 9 oz firm tofu, cubed
- 3 tablespoons low-sodium soy sauce
- 1 teaspoon sesame seeds
- 1 tablespoon sesame oil
- 1 cup spinach, chopped
- ¼ cup of water

Directions:

1. In the mixing bowl mix up soy sauce, and sesame oil.
2. Dip the tofu cubes in the soy sauce mixture and leave for 10 minutes to marinate.
3. Heat up a skillet and put the tofu cubes inside. Roast them for 1.5 minutes from each side.
4. Then add water, the remaining soy sauce mixture, and chopped spinach.
5. Close the lid and cook the meal for 5 minutes more.

Nutrition:

- 118 calories
- 8.5g protein
- 3.1g carbohydrates
- 8.6g fat
- 1.1g fiber
- 0mg cholesterol
- 406mg sodium

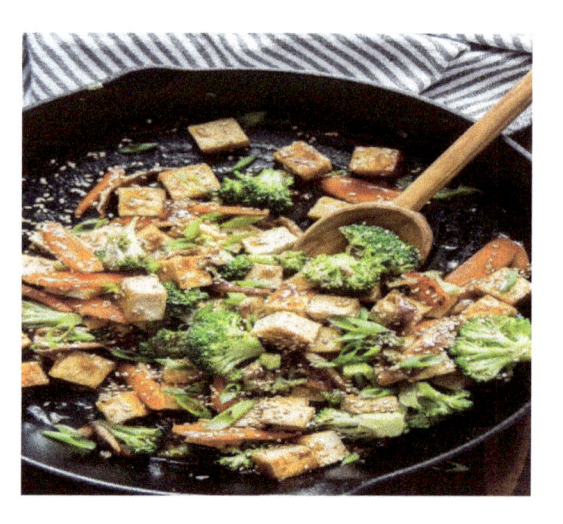

Mac Stuffed Sweet Potatoes

Preparation Time: 20 minutes

Cooking Time: 25 minutes

Servings: 2

Ingredients:

- 1 sweet potato
- ¼ cup whole-grain penne pasta
- 1 teaspoon tomato paste
- 1 teaspoon olive oil
- ¼ teaspoon minced garlic
- 1 tablespoon soy milk

Directions:

1. Cut the sweet potato in half and pierce it 3-4 times with the help of the fork.
2. Sprinkle the sweet potato halves with olive oil and bake in the preheated to 375F oven for 25-30 minutes or until the vegetables are tender.
3. Meanwhile, mix up penne pasta, tomato paste, minced garlic, and soy milk.
4. When the sweet potatoes are cooked, scoop out the vegetable meat and mix it up with a penne pasta mixture.
5. Fill the sweet potatoes with the pasta mixture.

Nutrition:

- 105 calories
- 2.7g protein
- 17.8g carbohydrates
- 2.8g fat
- 3g fiber
- 0mg cholesterol
- 28mg sodium

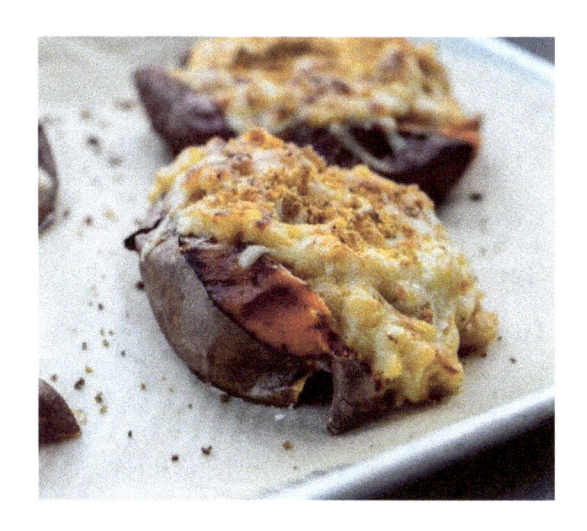

Tofu Tikka Masala

Preparation Time: 10 minutes

Cooking Time: 25 minutes

Servings: 2

Ingredients:

- 8 oz tofu, chopped
- ½ cup of soy milk
- 1 teaspoon garam masala
- 1 teaspoon olive oil
- 1 teaspoon ground paprika
- ½ cup tomatoes, chopped
- ½ onion, diced

Directions:

1. Heat up olive oil in the saucepan.
2. Add diced onion and cook it until light brown.
3. Then add tomatoes, ground paprika, and garam masala. Bring the mixture to a boil.
4. Add soy milk and stir well. Simmer it for 5 minutes.
5. Then add chopped tofu and cook the meal for 3 minutes.
6. Leave the cooked meal for 10 minutes to rest.

Nutrition:

- 155 calories
- 12.2g protein
- 20.7g carbohydrates
- 8.4g fat
- 2.9g fiber
- 0mg cholesterol
- 51mg sodium

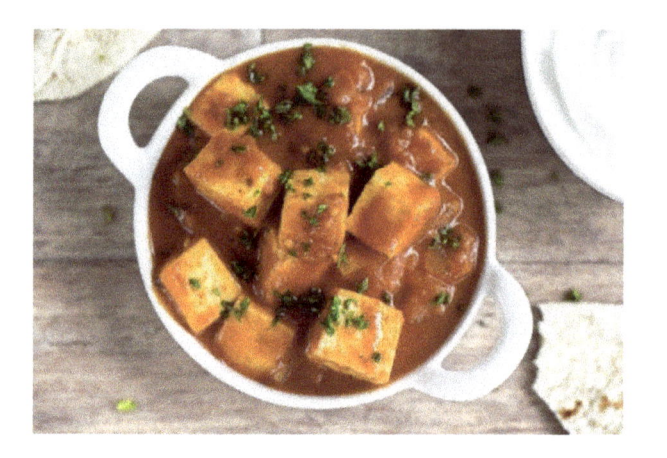

Tofu Parmigiana

Preparation Time: 15 minutes

Cooking Time: 8 minutes

Servings: 2

Ingredients:

- 6 oz firm tofu, roughly sliced
- 1 teaspoon coconut oil
- 1 teaspoon tomato sauce
- ½ teaspoon Italian seasonings

Directions:

1. In the mixing bowl, mix up, tomato sauce, and Italian seasonings.
2. Then brush the sliced tofu with the tomato mixture well and leave for 10 minutes to marinate.
3. Heat up coconut oil.
4. Then put the sliced tofu in the hot oil and roast it for 3 minutes per side or until tofu is golden brown.

Nutrition:

- 83 calories
- 7g protein
- 1.7g carbohydrates
- 6.2g fat
- 0.8 fiber
- 1mg cholesterol
- 24mg sodium

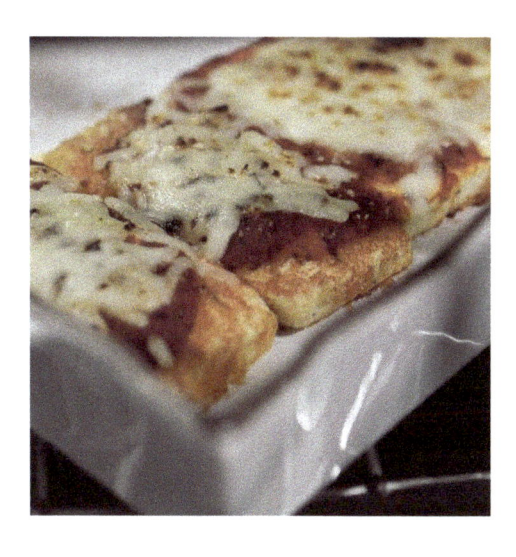

Mushroom Stroganoff

Preparation Time: 10 minutes

Cooking Time: 20 minutes

Servings: 2

Ingredients:

- 2 cups mushrooms, sliced
- 1 teaspoon whole-grain wheat flour
- 1 tablespoon coconut oil
- 1 onion, chopped
- 1 teaspoon dried thyme
- 1 garlic clove, diced
- 1 teaspoon ground black pepper
- ½ cup of soy milk

Directions:

- Heat up coconut oil in the saucepan.
- Add mushrooms and onion and cook them for 10 minutes. Stir the vegetables from time to time.
- After this, sprinkle them with ground black pepper, thyme, and garlic.
- Add soy milk and bring the mixture to a boil.
- Then add flour and stir it well until homogenous.
- Cook the mushroom stroganoff until it thickens.

Nutrition:

- 70 calories
- 2.6g protein
- 6.9g carbohydrates
- 4.1g fat
- 1.5g fiber
- 0mg cholesterol
- 19mg sodium

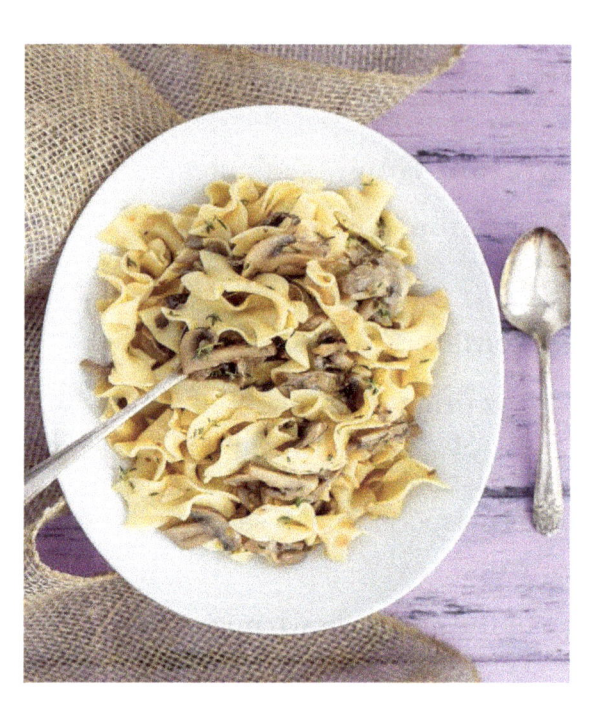

Eggplant Croquettes

Preparation Time: 15 minutes

Cooking Time: 5 minutes

Servings: 2

Ingredients:

- 1 eggplant, peeled, boiled
- 2 potatoes, mashed
- 2 tablespoons almond meal
- 1 teaspoon chili pepper
- 1 tablespoon coconut oil
- 1 tablespoon olive oil
- ¼ teaspoon ground nutmeg

Directions:

1. Blend the eggplant until smooth.
2. Then mix it up with mashed potato, chili pepper, coconut oil, and ground nutmeg.
3. Make the croquettes from the eggplant mixture.
4. Heat up olive oil in the skillet.
5. Put the croquettes in the hot oil and cook them for 2 minutes per side or until they are light brown.

Nutrition:

- 180 calories
- 3.6g protein
- 24.3g carbohydrates
- 8.8g fat
- 7.1g fiber
- 0mg cholesterol
- 9mg sodium

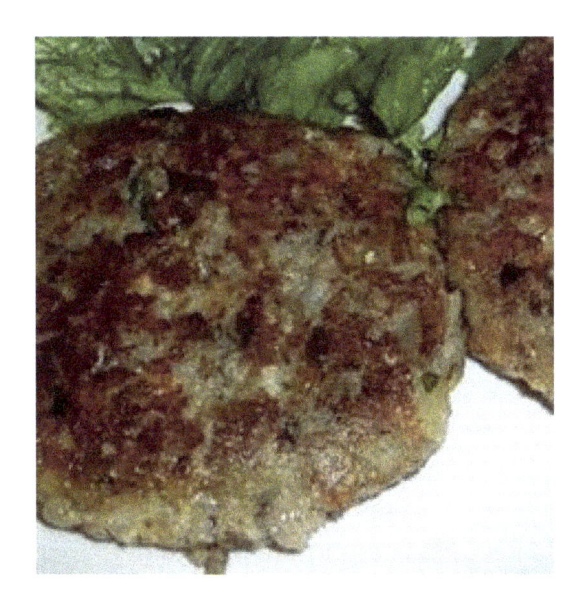

Stuffed Portobello

Preparation Time: 10 minutes

Cooking Time: 20 minutes

Servings: 2

Ingredients:

- 4 Portobello mushroom caps
- ½ zucchini, grated
- 1 tomato, diced
- 1 teaspoon olive oil
- ½ teaspoon dried parsley
- ¼ teaspoon minced garlic

Directions:

1. In the mixing bowl, mix up diced tomato, grated zucchini, dried parsley, and minced garlic.
2. Then fill the mushroom caps with zucchini mixture and transfer to the lined baking paper tray.
3. Bake the vegetables for 20 minutes or until they are soft.

Nutrition:

- 24 calories
- 1.2g protein
- 2.9g carbohydrates
- 1.3g fat
- 0.9g fiber
- 0mg cholesterol
- 5mg sodium

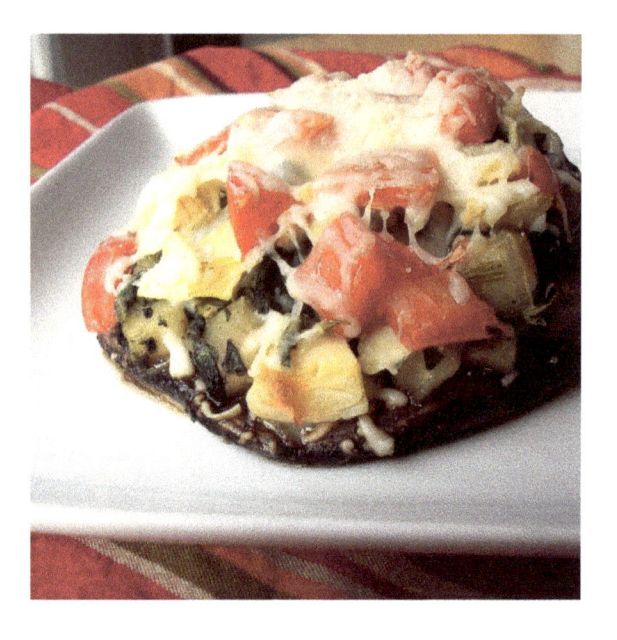

Chile Rellenos

Preparation Time: 10 minutes

Cooking Time: 30 minutes

Servings: 2

Ingredients:

- 2 chili peppers
- 2 oz vegan Mozzarella cheese, shredded
- 2 oz tomato puree
- 1 tablespoon coconut oil
- 2 tablespoons whole-grain wheat flour
- 1 tablespoon potato starch
- ¼ cup of water
- ½ teaspoon chili flakes

Directions:

1. Bake the chili peppers for 15 minutes in the preheated to 375F oven.
2. Meanwhile, pour tomato puree into the saucepan.
3. Add chili flakes and bring the mixture to boil. Remove it from the heat.
4. After this, mix up potato starch, flour, and water.
5. When the chili peppers are cooked, make the cuts in them and remove the seeds.
6. Then fill the peppers with shredded cheese and secure the cuts with toothpicks.
7. Heat up coconut oil in the skillet.
8. Dip the chili peppers in the flour mixture and roast in the coconut oil until they are golden brown.
9. Sprinkle the cooked chilies with the tomato puree mixture.

Nutrition:

- 187 calories
- 4.2g protein
- 16g carbohydrates
- 12g fat
- 3.7g fiber
- 0mg cholesterol
- 122mg sodium

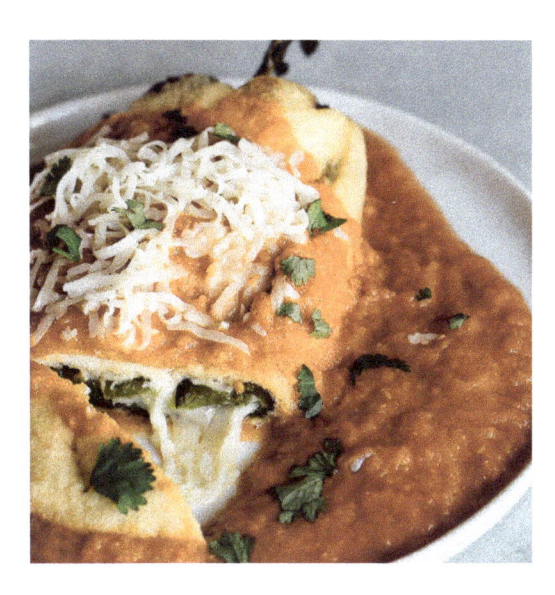

Garbanzo Stir Fry

Preparation Time: 10 minutes

Cooking Time: 30 minutes

Ingredients:

Servings: 2

- 1 cup garbanzo beans, cooked
- 1 zucchini, diced
- 5 oz cremini mushrooms, chopped
- 1 tablespoon coconut oil
- 1 teaspoon ground black pepper
- 1 tablespoon fresh parsley, chopped
- 1 tablespoon lemon juice

Directions:

1. Heat up coconut oil in the saucepan.
2. Add mushrooms and roast them for 10 minutes.
3. Then add zucchini and cooked garbanzo beans. Stir the ingredients well and cook them for 10 minutes more.
4. After this, sprinkle the vegetables with ground black pepper and lemon juice. Cook the meal for 5 minutes.
5. Add parsley and mix it up. Cook it for 5 minutes more.

Nutrition:

- 231 calories
- 11.3g protein
- 33.9g carbohydrates
- 6.6g fat
- 9.6g fiber
- 0mg cholesterol
- 21mg sodium

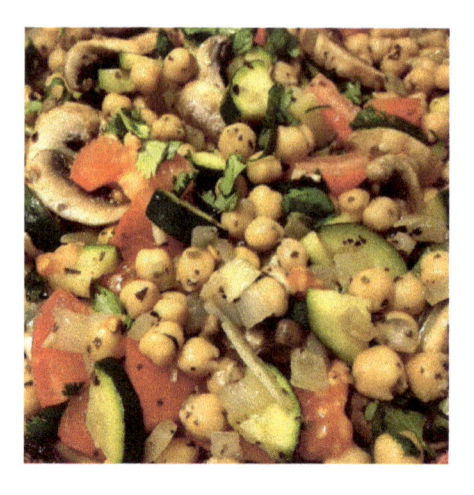

CHAPTER 6:

Fish & Seafood

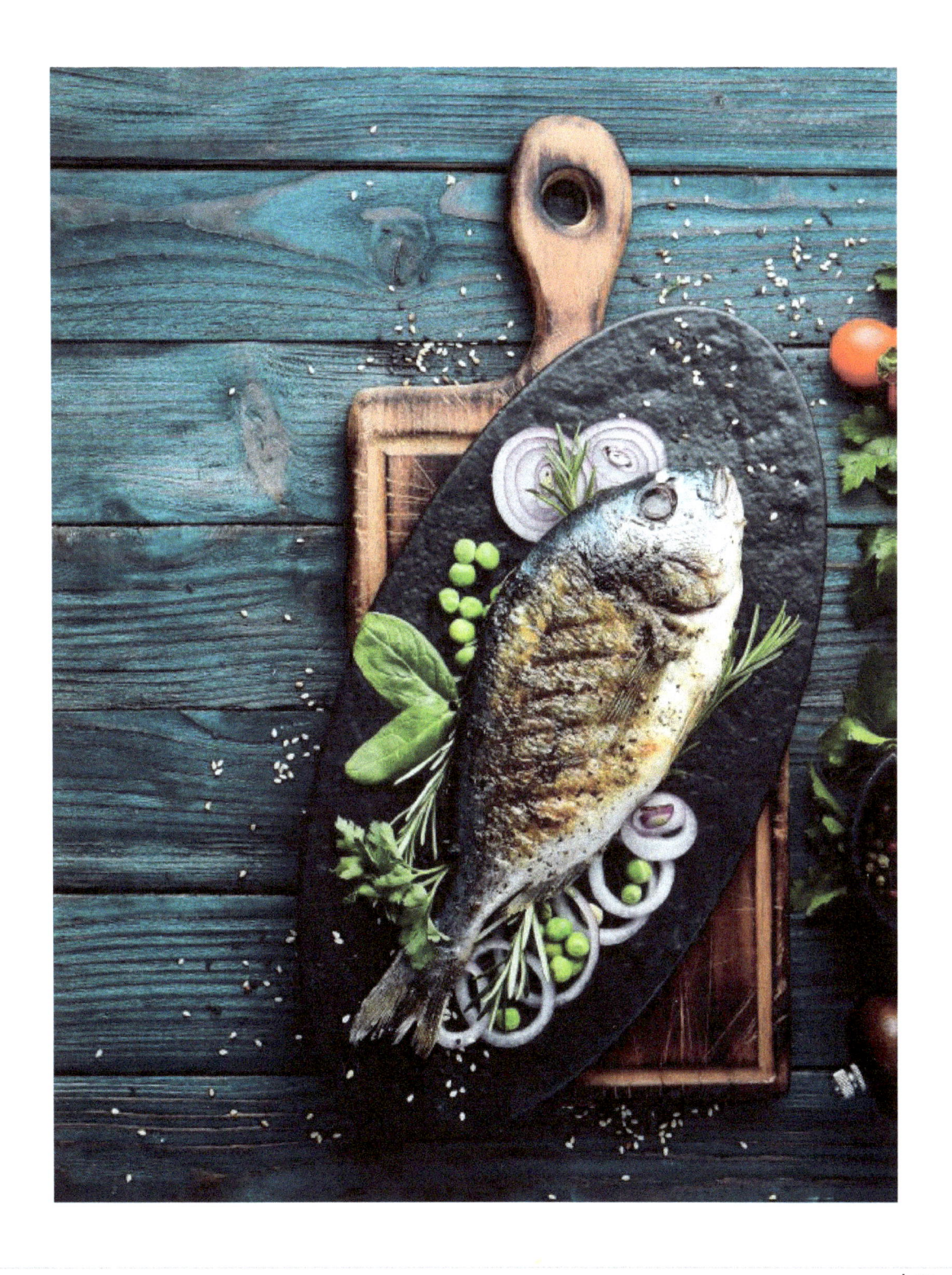

Halibut with Tomato, Basil, and Oregano Salsa

Preparation Time: 20 minutes

Cooking Time: 15 minutes

Servings: 2

Ingredients:

- Tomatoes - 2 diced
- Fresh basil - 2 tablespoons chopped
- Fresh oregano - 1 teaspoon chopped
- Garlic - 1 tablespoon minced
- Extra virgin olive oil - 2 teaspoons
- Halibut filets -4 ounces each
- Parmesan cheese - optional

Directions:

1. Preheat the oven to 350 °F (150 °C).
2. Lightly coat a glass 9 x 13-inch baking dish with cooking spray.
3. In a mixer, combine the tomato, basil, oregano, and garlic on chopping speed. Add the olive oil and chop for another minute to blend.
4. Arrange the halibut fillets in the baking dish. Pour the tomato mixture over the fish evenly. Place in the oven and bake for about 10 to 15 minutes.
5. Transfer to individual plates and spoon some of the tomato sauce over each fillet then serve immediately.
6. Sprinkle a little parmesan cheese over the top for an added kick of flavor.

Nutrition:

- Total fat 5 g
- Calories 160
- Protein 24 g
- Cholesterol 36 mg
- Total carbohydrate 3 g
- Dietary fiber 1 g
- Sodium 65 mg

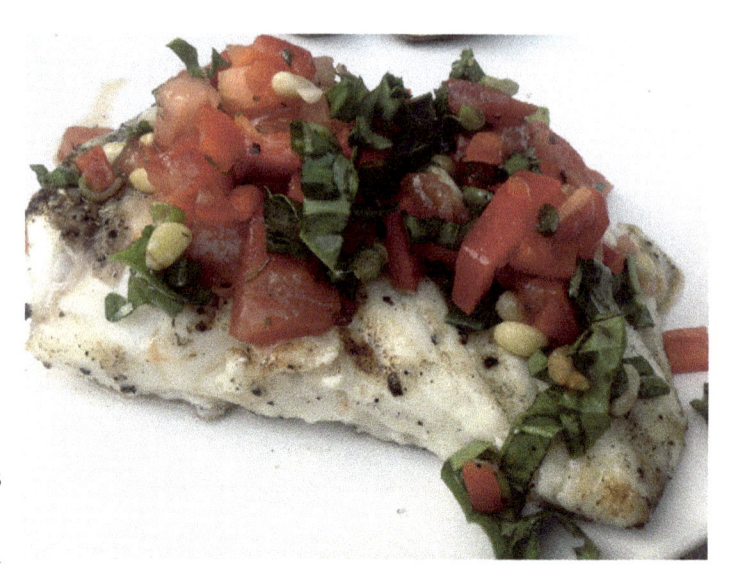

Roasted Salmon with Chives and Tarragon

Preparation Time: 20 minutes

Cooking Time: 12 minutes

Servings: 2

Ingredients:

- Organic salmon with skin - 2 - 5 ounce pieces
- Extra virgin olive oil - 2 teaspoons
- Chives - 1 tablespoon chopped
- Fresh tarragon leaves - 1 teaspoon
- Cooking spray

Directions:

1. Preheat oven to 475 °F (250 °C).
2. Line a baking sheet with foil and light cooking spray.
3. Rub salmon with 2 teaspoons of extra virgin olive oil.
4. Roast skin side down about 12 minutes or until fish is thoroughly cooked.
5. Use a metal spatula to lift the salmon off the skin. Place salmon on the serving plate. Discard skin. Sprinkle salmon with herbs and serve.

Nutrition:

- Sodium 62 mg
- Total fat 14 g
- Cholesterol 78 mg
- Protein 28 g
- Calories 241
- Total carbohydrate 3.2 g

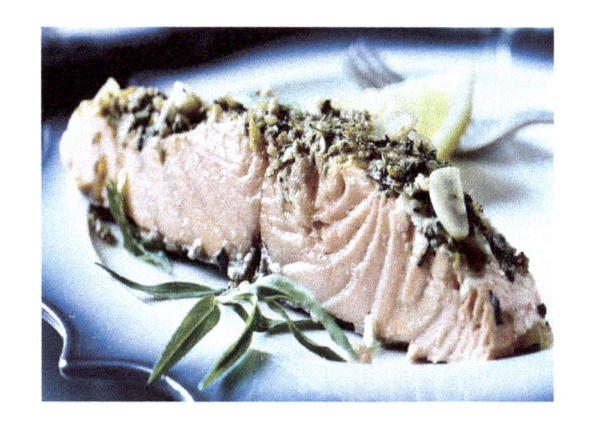

Grilled Shrimp Salad with Orange Vinaigrette

Preparation Time: 10 minutes

Cooking Time: 6 minutes

Servings: 2

Ingredients:

- 1 orange, juiced
- 1 lime, juiced
- 1 tsp fresh mint, chopped
- 1/2-lb. tail-on shrimps
- 1 small red onion, quartered
- 2 cups packed spinach leaves
- 1 avocado, peeled, seeded, and sliced
- 1 cup cherry tomatoes, sliced in half
- 1 orange, cut into segments

Directions:

1. In a small bowl, whisk well orange juice, lime juice, and mint.
2. In a medium bowl add shrimp a tbsp of the orange vinaigrette. Toss well to coat.
3. Skewer shrimps and red onion. Grill on preheated 400oF oven or grill for 4 minutes per side. Remove from grill and set aside to cool.
4. Evenly divide between two bowls the spinach leaves, avocado, cherry tomatoes, red onion, grilled shrimp, grilled onions, and orange segments.
5. Drizzle with vinaigrette, toss well to coat.
6. Serve and enjoy.

Nutrition:

- Calories: 351
- Protein: 27.7g
- Carbs: 31.0g
- Fat: 15.8g
- Saturated Fat: 2.3g
- Sodium: 172mg

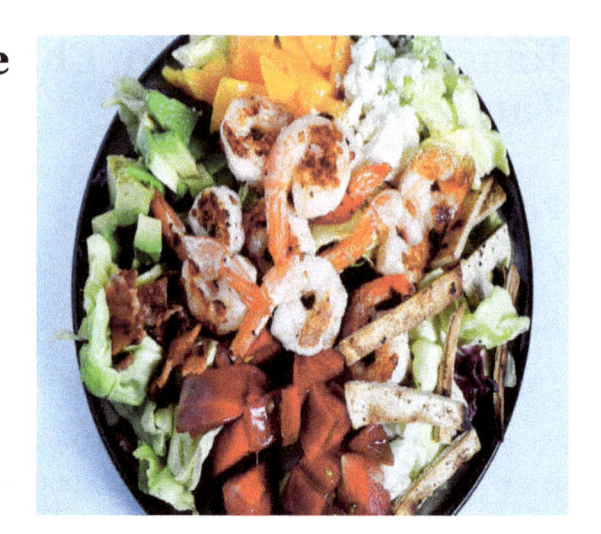

Halibut with Radish Slices

Preparation Time: 10 minutes

Cooking Time: 6 minutes

Servings: 2

Ingredients:

- 4 halibut fillets, boneless
- 1 cup radishes, sliced
- 1 tablespoon apple cider vinegar
- ¼ teaspoon ground coriander
- 1 tablespoon olive oil
- 1 teaspoon low-fat cream cheese

Directions:

1. Sprinkle the fish fillets with apple cider vinegar, ground coriander, and olive oil.
2. Then grill the halibut in the preheated to 385F grill for 3 minutes per side.
3. Transfer the fish to the plates and top with sliced radish and cream cheese.

Nutrition:

- 356 calories
- 60.8g protein
- 1g carbohydrates
- 10.5g fat
- 0.5g fiber
- 94mg cholesterol
- 170mg sodium

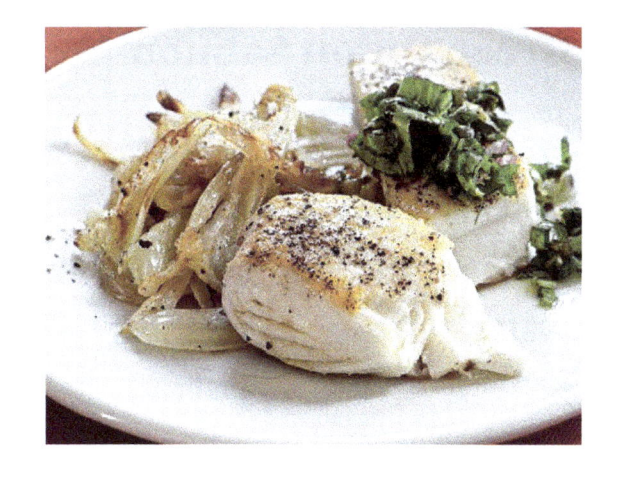

Green Onion Salmon

Preparation Time: 10 minutes

Cooking Time: 10 minutes

Servings: 2

Ingredients:

4 green olives, pitted, sliced

2 oz green onions, blended

½ teaspoon chili flakes

¼ teaspoon ground black pepper

3 tablespoons avocado oil

4 salmon fillets, skinless and boneless

1 oz parsley, chopped

Directions:

1. Blend together green onions, chili flakes, ground black pepper, avocado oil, and parsley.
2. Then rub the salmon fillets with green onion mixture and transfer them to the preheated skillet.
3. Cook it for 4 minutes per side.
4. Top the cooked fish with sliced olives.

Nutrition:

- 272 calories
- 35.1g protein
- 3.2g carbohydrates
- 13.4g fat
- 1.1g fiber
- 78mg cholesterol
- 375mg sodium

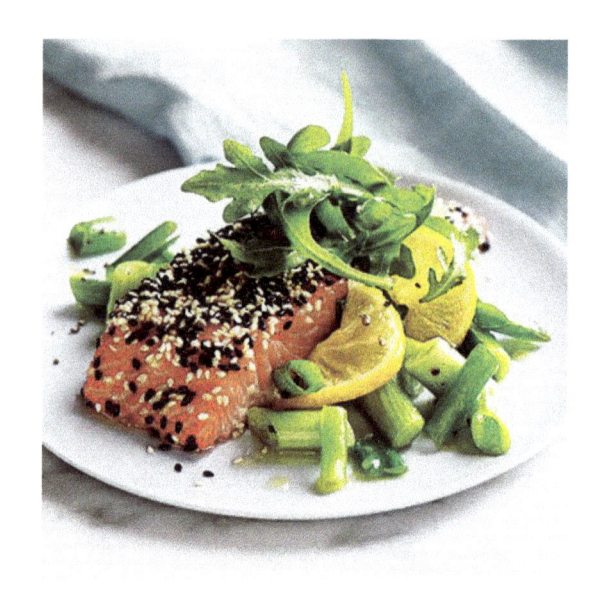

Broccoli and Cod Mash

Preparation Time: 10 minutes

Cooking Time: 20 minutes

Servings: 1

Ingredients:

- 2 cups broccoli, chopped
- 4 cod fillets, boneless, chopped
- 1 white onion, chopped
- 2 tablespoons olive oil
- 1 cup of water
- 1 tablespoon low-fat cream cheese
- ½ teaspoon ground black pepper

Directions:

1. Roast the cod in the saucepan with olive oil for 1 minute per side.
2. Then add all remaining ingredients except cream cheese and boil the meal for 18 minutes.
3. After this, drain water, add cream cheese, and stir the meal well.

Nutrition:

- 186 calories
- 21.8g protein
- 5.8g carbohydrates
- 9.1g fat
- 1.8g fiber
- 43mg cholesterol
- 105mg sodium

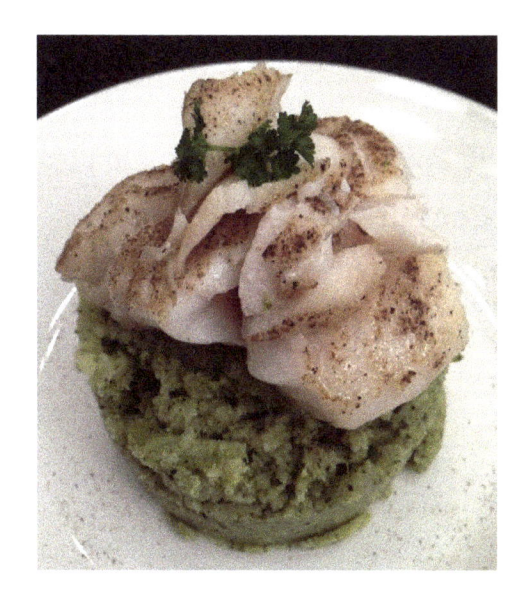

Greek Style Salmon

Preparation Time: 10 minutes

Cooking Time: 10 minutes

Servings: 2

Ingredients:

- 4 medium salmon fillets, skinless and boneless
- 1 tablespoon lemon juice
- 1 tablespoon dried oregano
- 1 teaspoon dried thyme
- ¼ teaspoon onion powder
- 1 tablespoon olive oil

Directions:

1. Heat up olive oil in the skillet.
2. Sprinkle the salmon with dried oregano, thyme, onion powder, and lemon juice.
3. Put the fish in the skillet and cook for 4 minutes per side.

Nutrition:

- 271 calories
- 34.7g protein
- 1.1g carbohydrates
- 14.7g fat
- 0.6g fiber
- 78mg cholesterol
- 80mg sodium

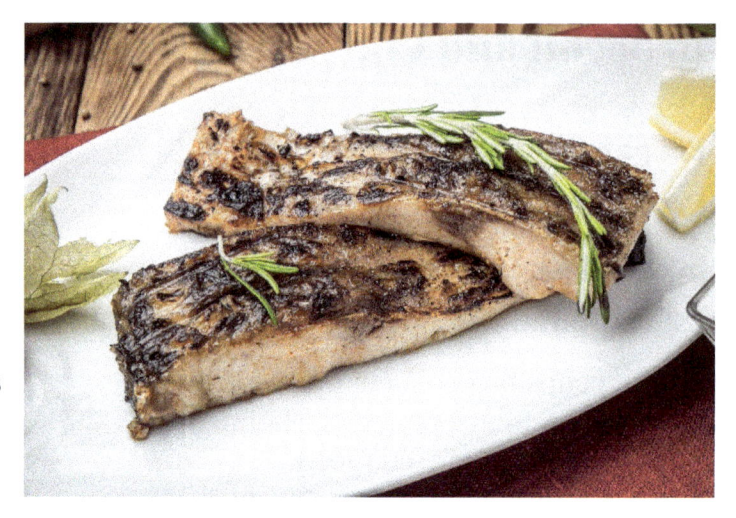

Spicy Ginger Seabass

Preparation Time: 5 minutes

Cooking Time: 10 minutes

Servings: 2

Ingredients:

- 1 tablespoon ginger, grated
- 2 tablespoons sesame oil
- ¼ teaspoon chili powder
- 4 sea bass fillets, boneless
- 1 tablespoon margarine

Directions:

1. Heat up sesame oil and margarine in the skillet.
2. Add chili powder and ginger.
3. Then add seabass and cook the fish for 3 minutes per side.
4. Then close the lid and simmer the fish for 3 minutes over low heat.

Nutrition:

- 216 calories
- 24g protein
- 1.1g carbohydrates
- 12.3g fat
- 0.2g fiber
- 54mg cholesterol
- 123mg sodium

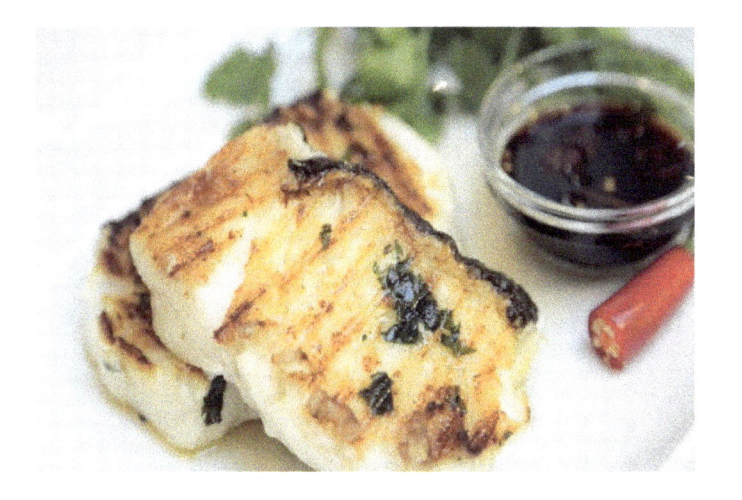

Yogurt Shrimps

Preparation Time: 5 minutes

Cooking Time: 10 minutes

Servings: 2

Ingredients:

- 1 pound shrimp, peeled
- 1 tablespoon margarine
- ¼ cup low-fat yogurt
- 1 teaspoon lemon zest, grated
- 1 chili pepper, chopped

Directions:

1. Melt the margarine in the skillet, add chili pepper, and roast it for 1 minute.
2. Then add shrimps and lemon zest.
3. Roast the shrimps for 2 minutes per side.
4. After this, add yogurt, stir the shrimps well and cook for 5 minutes.

Nutrition:

- 137 calories
- 21.4g protein
- 2.4g carbohydrates
- 4g fat
- 0.1g fiber
- 192mg cholesterol
- 257mg sodium

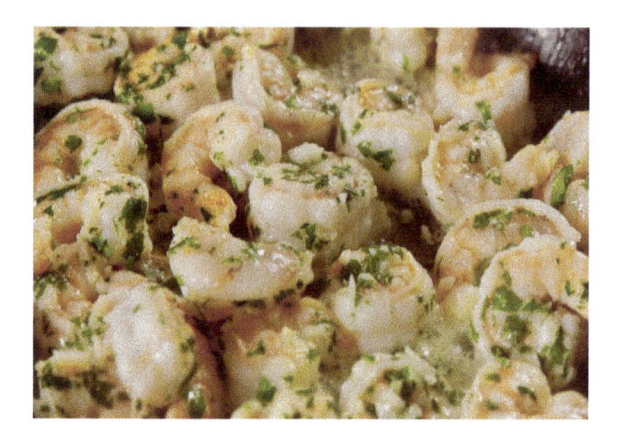

Aromatic Salmon with Fennel Seeds

Preparation Time: 8 minutes

Cooking Time: 10 minutes

Servings: 2

Ingredients:

- 4 medium salmon fillets, skinless and boneless
- 1 tablespoon fennel seeds
- 2 tablespoons olive oil
- 1 tablespoon lemon juice
- 1 tablespoon water

Directions:

1. Heat up olive oil in the skillet.
2. Add fennel seeds and roast them for 1 minute.
3. Add salmon fillets and sprinkle with lemon juice.
4. Add water and roast the fish for 4 minutes per side over medium heat.

Nutrition:

- 301 calories
- 4.8g protein
- 0.8g carbohydrates
- 18.2g fat
- 0.6g fiber
- 78mg cholesterol
- 81mg sodium

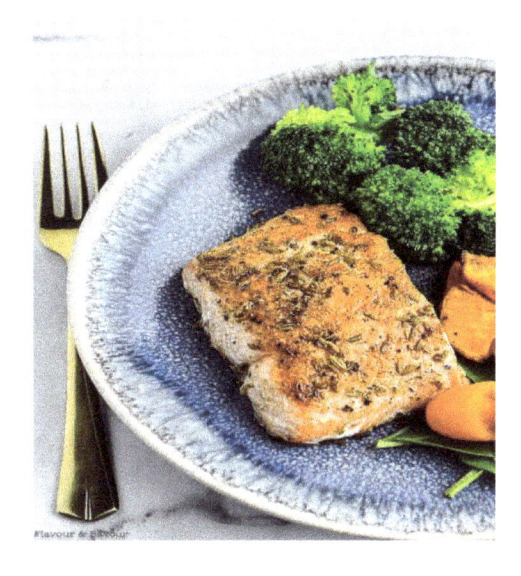

Shrimp Quesadillas

Preparation Time: 16 minutes

Cooking Time: 5 minutes

Servings: 2

Ingredients:

- Two whole wheat tortillas
- ½ tsp. ground cumin
- 4 cilantro leaves
- 3 oz. diced cooked shrimp
- 1 de-seeded plump tomato
- ¾ c. grated non-fat mozzarella cheese
- ¼ c. diced red onion

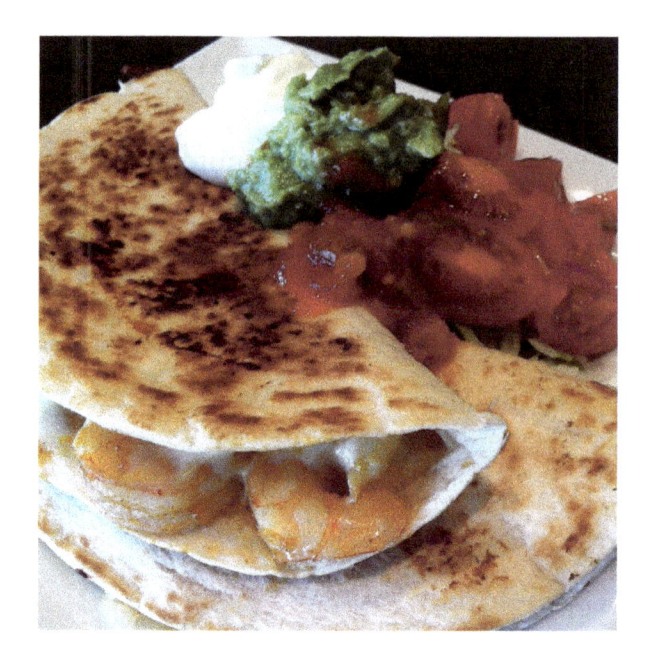

Directions:

1. In a medium bowl, combine the grated mozzarella cheese and the warm, cooked shrimp. Add the ground cumin, red onion, and tomato. Mix. Spread the mixture evenly on the tortillas.
2. Heat a non-stick frying pan. Place the tortillas in the pan, then heat until they crisp.
3. Add the cilantro leaves. Fold over the tortillas.
4. Press down for 1 – 2 minutes. Slice the tortillas into wedges.
5. Serve immediately.

Nutrition:

- Calories: 99
- Fat: 9 g
- Carbs: 7.2 g
- Protein: 59 g
- Sugars: 4 g
- Sodium: 500 mg

The OG Tuna Sandwich

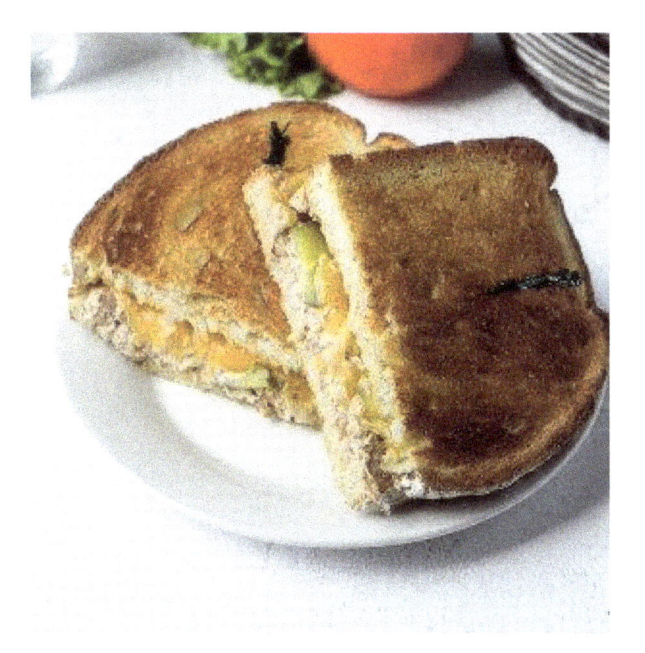

Preparation Time: 15 minutes

Cooking Time: 5 minutes

Servings: 2

Ingredients:

- 30 g olive oil
- 1 peeled and diced medium cucumber
- 2 ½ g pepper
- 4 whole-wheat bread slices
- 85 g diced onion
- 2 ½ g salt
- 1 can flavored tuna
- 85 g shredded spinach

Directions:

1. Grab your blender and add the spinach, tuna, onion, oil, salt, and pepper, and pulse for about 10 to 20 seconds.
2. In the meantime, toast your bread and add your diced cucumber to a bowl, which you can pour your tuna mixture in. Carefully mix and add the mixture to the bread once toasted.
3. Slice in half and serve, while storing the remaining mixture in the fridge.

Nutrition:

- Calories: 302
- Fat: 5.8 g
- Carbs: 36.62 g
- Protein: 28 g
- Sugars: 3.22 g
- Sodium: 445 mg

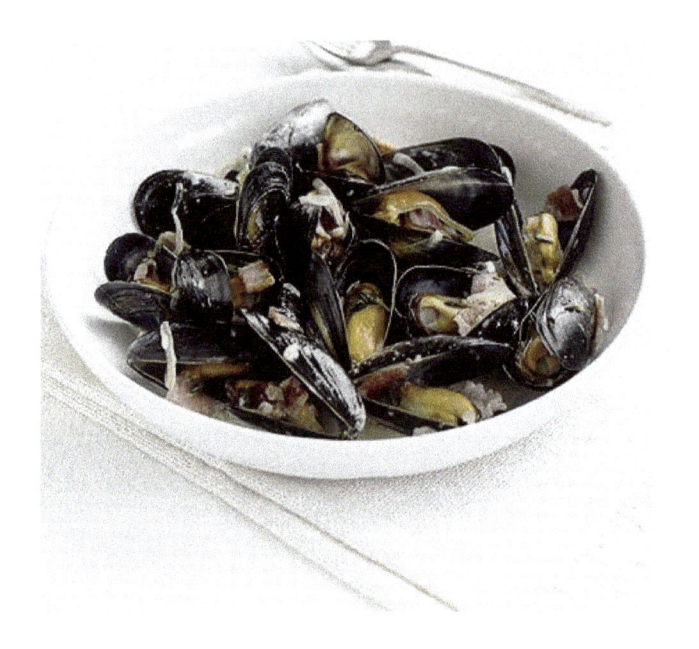

Easy To Make Mussels

Preparation Time: 10 minutes

Cooking Time: 10 minutes

Servings: 2

Ingredients:

- 2 lbs. cleaned mussels
- 4 minced garlic cloves
- 2 chopped shallots
- Lemon and parsley
- 2 tbsps. Butter
- ½ c. broth
- ½ c. white wine

Directions:

1. Clean the mussels and remove the beard.
2. Discard any mussels that do not close when tapped against a hard surface.
3. Set your pot to Sauté mode and add chopped onion and butter.
4. Stir and sauté onions.
5. Add garlic and cook for 1 minute.
6. Add broth and wine.
7. Lock up the lid and cook for 5 minutes on HIGH pressure.
8. Release the pressure naturally over 10 minutes.
9. Serve with a sprinkle of parsley and enjoy!

Nutrition:

- Calories: 286
- Fat: 14 g
- Carbs: 12 g
- Protein: 28 g
- Sugars: 0 g
- Sodium: 314 mg

Chili-Rubbed Tilapia with Asparagus & Lemon

Preparation Time: 10 minutes

Cooking Time: 10 minutes

Servings: 2

Ingredients:

- 3 tbsps. lemon juice
- 2 tbsps. chili powder
- 2 tbsps. extra-virgin olive oil
- ½ tsp. divided salt
- 2 lbs. trimmed asparagus
- ½ tsp. garlic powder
- 1 lb. tilapia fillets

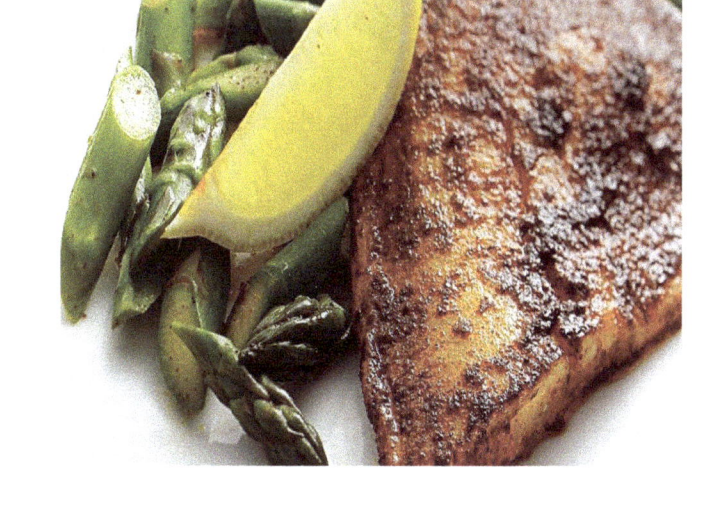

Directions:

1. Bring 1 inch of water to a boil in a large saucepan. Put asparagus in a steamer basket, place in the pan, cover, and steam until tender-crisp, about 4 minutes.
2. Transfer to a large plate, spreading out to cool.
3. Combine chili powder, garlic powder, and ¼ teaspoon salt on a plate. Dredge fillets in the spice mixture to coat. Heat oil in a large nonstick skillet over medium-high heat. Add the fish and cook until just opaque in the center, gently turning halfway, and 5 to 7 minutes total.
4. Divide among 4 plates. Immediately add lemon juice, the remaining ¼ teaspoon salt, and asparagus to the pan and cook, stirring constantly, until the asparagus is coated and heated through, about 2 minutes.
5. Serve the asparagus with the fish.

Nutrition:

- Calories: 211
- Fat: 10 g
- Carbs: 8 g
- Protein: 26 g
- Sugars: 0.4 g
- Sodium: 375.7 mg

Parmesan-Crusted Fish

Preparation Time: 5 minutes

Cooking Time: 7 minutes

Servings: 2

Ingredients:

- ¾ tsp. ground ginger
- 1/3 c. panko bread crumbs
- Mixed fresh salad greens
- ¼ c. finely shredded parmesan cheese
- 1 tbsp. butter
- 4 skinless cod fillets
- 3 c. julienned carrots

Directions:

1. Preheat oven to 450 ₀F. Lightly coat a baking sheet with nonstick cooking spray.
2. Rinse and pat dry fish; place on the baking sheet. Season with salt and pepper.
3. In a small bowl stir together crumbs and cheese; sprinkle on fish.
4. Bake, uncovered, 4 to 6 minutes for each 1/2-inch thickness of fish, until crumbs are golden and fish flakes easily when tested with a fork.
5. Meanwhile, in a large skillet bring 1/2 cup water to boiling; add carrots. Reduce heat.
6. Cook, covered, for 5 minutes. Uncover; cook 2 minutes more. Add butter and ginger; toss.
7. Serve fish and carrots with greens.

Nutrition:

- Calories: 216.4
- Fat: 10.1 g
- Carbs: 1.3 g
- Protein: 29.0 g
- Sugars: 0.1 g
- Sodium: 428.3 mg

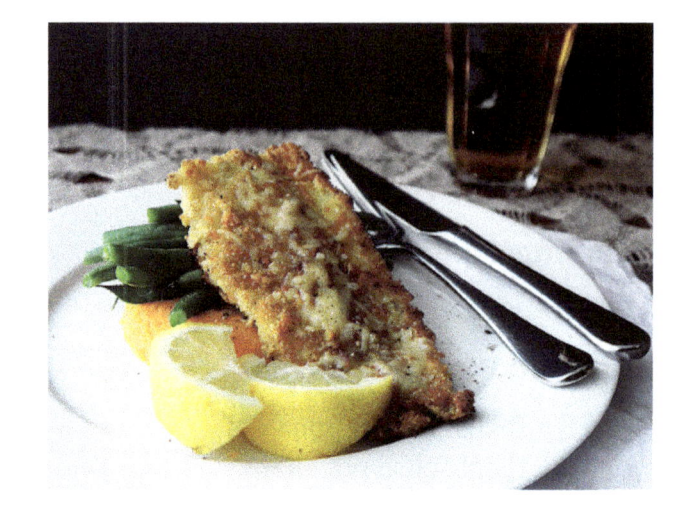

Lemon Swordfish

Preparation Time: 10 minutes

Cooking Time: 25 minutes

Servings: 2

Ingredients:

- 18 oz swordfish fillets
- 1 tablespoon margarine
- 1 teaspoon lemon zest
- 3 tablespoons lemon juice
- 1 teaspoon ground black pepper
- 2 tablespoons olive oil
- ½ teaspoon minced garlic

Directions:

1. Cut the fish into 4 servings.
2. After this, in the mixing bowl, mix up lemon zest, lemon juice, ground black pepper, and olive oil. Add minced garlic.
3. Rub the fish fillets with lemon mixture.
4. Grease the baking pan with margarine and arrange the swordfish fillets.
5. Bake the fish for 25 minutes at 390F.

Nutrition:

- 288 calories
- 32.6g protein
- 0.8g carbohydrates
- 16.5g fat
- 0.2g fiber
- 64mg cholesterol
- 183mg sodium

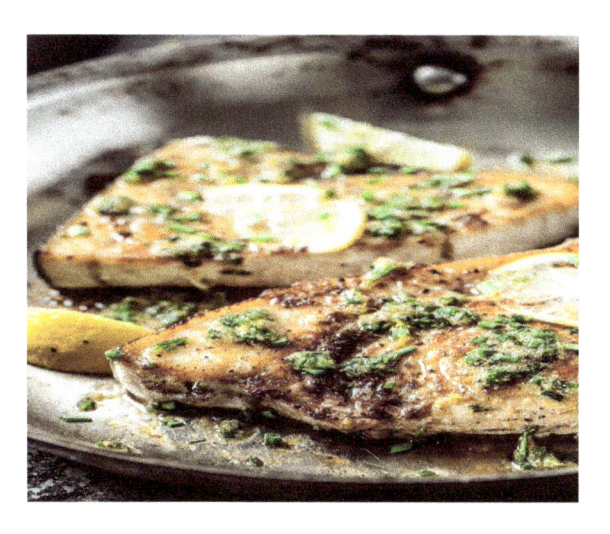

Spiced Scallops

Preparation Time: 10 minutes

Cooking Time: 5 minutes

Servings: 2

Ingredients:

- 1-pound scallops
- 1 teaspoon Cajun seasonings
- 1 tablespoon olive oil

Directions:

1. Rub the scallops with Cajun seasonings.
2. Heat up olive oil in the skillet.
3. Add scallops and cook them for 2 minutes per each side.

Nutrition:

- 130 calories
- 19g protein
- 2.7g carbohydrates
- 4.4g fat
- 0g fiber
- 37mg cholesterol
- 195mg sodium

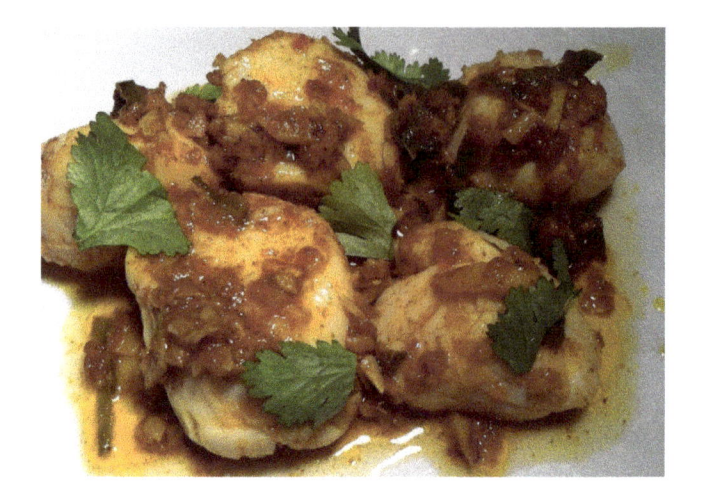

Shrimp Puttanesca

Preparation Time: 5 minutes

Cooking Time: 20 minutes

Servings: 2

Ingredients:

- 5 oz shrimps, peeled
- 1 teaspoon chili flakes
- ½ onion, diced
- 1 tablespoon coconut oil
- 1 teaspoon garlic, diced
- 1 cup tomatoes, chopped
- ¼ cup olives, sliced
- ¼ cup of water

Directions:

1. Heat up coconut oil in the saucepan.
2. Add shrimps and chili flakes. Cook the shrimps for 4 minutes.
3. Stir them well and add diced onion, garlic, tomatoes, olives, and water.
4. Close the lid and sauté the meal for 15 minutes.

Nutrition:

- 128 calories
- 11.7g protein
- 5.8g carbohydrates
- 6.7g fat
- 1.5g fiber
- 100mg cholesterol
- 217mg sodium

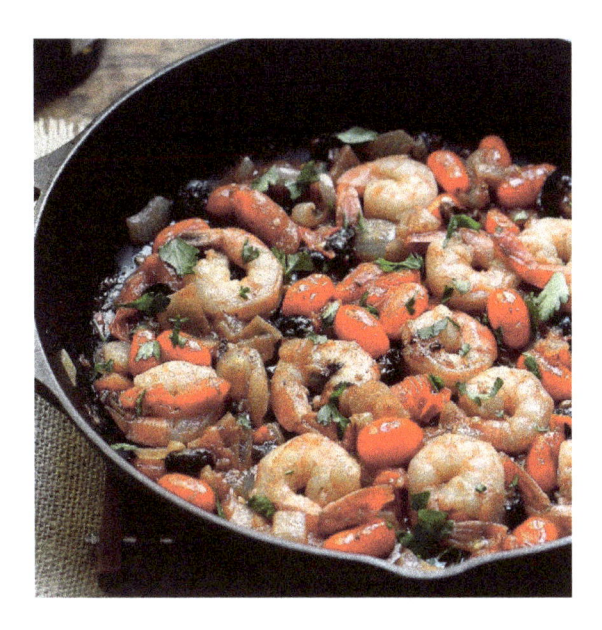

Curry Snapper

Preparation Time: 10 minutes

Cooking Time: 15 minutes

Servings: 2

Ingredients:

- 1-pound snapper fillet, chopped
- 1 teaspoon curry powder
- 1 cup celery stalk, chopped
- ½ cup low-fat yogurt
- ¼ cup of water
- 1 tablespoon olive oil

Directions:

1. Roast the snapper fillet in olive oil for 2 minutes per side.
2. Then add celery stalk, curry powder, low-fat yogurt, and water.
3. Stir the fish until you get the homogenous texture.
4. Close the lid and simmer the fish for 10 minutes on medium heat.

Nutrition:

- 195 calories
- 29.5g protein
- 3.2g carbohydrates
- 5.9g fat
- 0.6g fiber
- 52mg cholesterol
- 105mg sodium

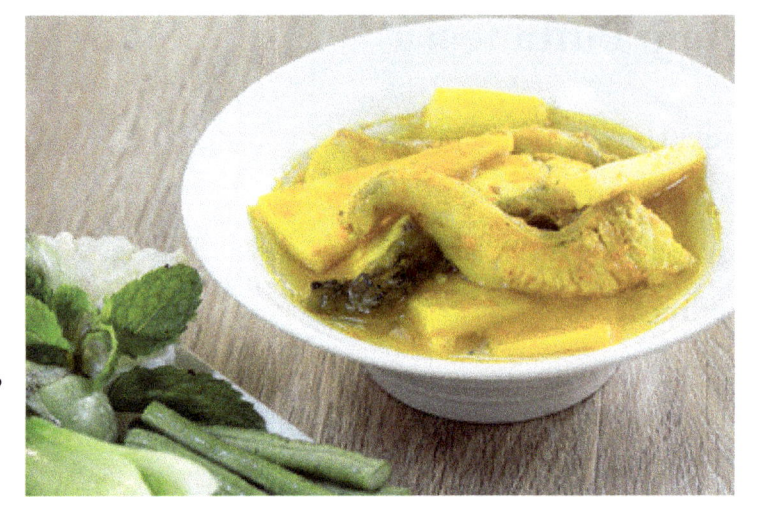

Grouper with Tomato Sauce

Preparation Time: 10 minutes

Cooking Time: 15 minutes

Servings: 2

Ingredients:

- 12 oz grouper, chopped
- 2 cups grape tomatoes, chopped
- 1 chili pepper, chopped
- 1 tablespoon margarine
- 1 teaspoon ground coriander

Directions:

1. Toss the margarine in the saucepan.
2. Add chopped grouper and sprinkle it with ground coriander.
3. Roast the fish for 2 minutes per side.
4. Then add grape tomatoes and chili pepper.
5. Stir the ingredients well and close the lid.
6. Cook the meal for 10 minutes on low heat.

Nutrition:

- 285 calories
- 43.9g protein
- 7.2g carbohydrates
- 8.3g fat
- 2.2g fiber
- 80mg cholesterol
- 166mg sodium

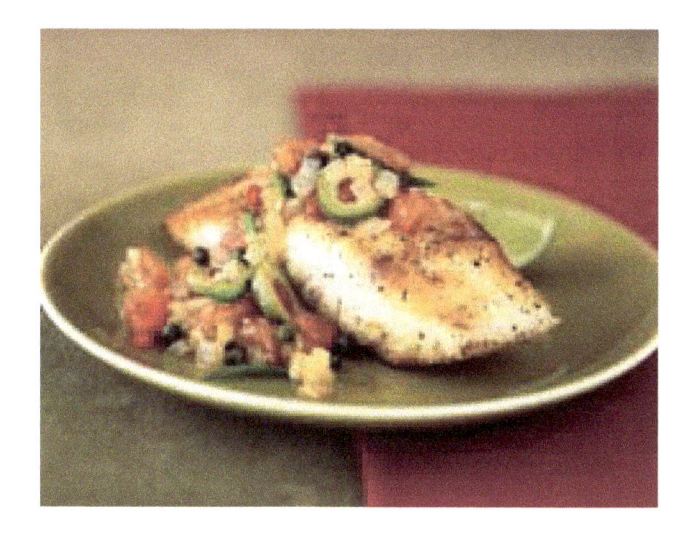

Braised Seabass

Preparation Time: 8 minutes

Cooking Time: 28 minutes

Servings: 2

Ingredients:

- 10 oz seabass fillet
- 1 cup tomatoes, chopped
- 1 yellow onion, sliced
- 1 tablespoon avocado oil
- 1 teaspoon ground black pepper

Directions:

1. Heat up olive oil in the skillet.
2. Add seabass fillet and roast it for 4 minutes per side.
3. Then remove the fish from the skillet and add sliced onion.
4. Cook it for 2 minutes.
5. After this, add tomatoes, and ground black pepper.
6. Bring the mixture to a boil.
7. Add cooked seabass and close the lid.
8. Cook the meal for 15 minutes.

Nutrition:

- 285 calories
- 27.7g protein
- 9.7g carbohydrates
- 15.3g fat
- 3.8g fiber
- 0mg cholesterol
- 8mg sodium

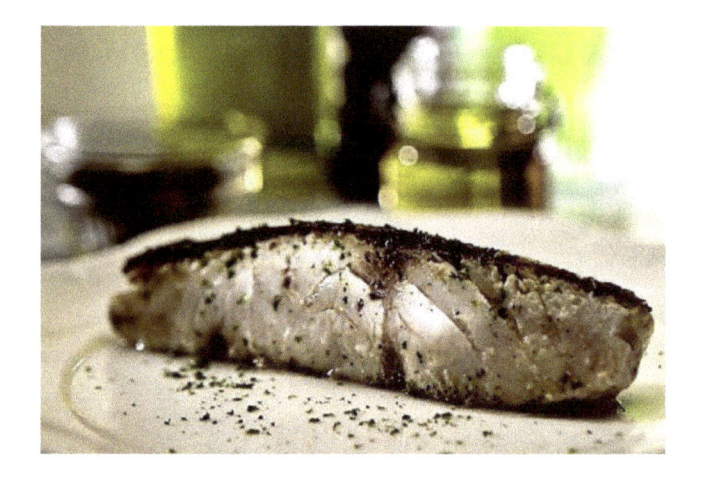

CHAPTER 7:

Pork & Beef

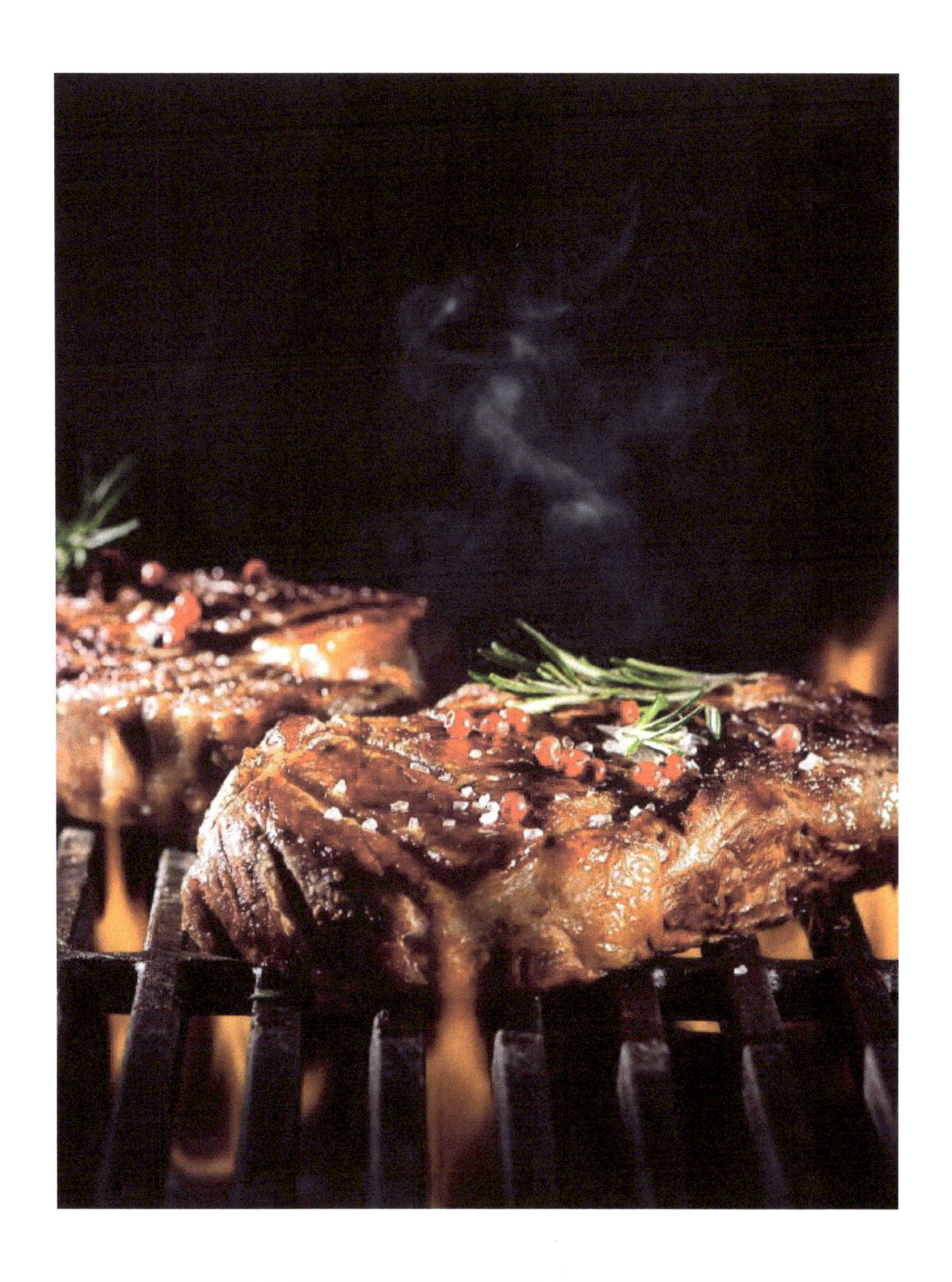

Beef Stroganoff

Preparation Time: 50 minutes

Cooking Time: 45 minutes

Servings: 2

Ingredients:

- One cup sour cream, fat-free
- Four cloves garlic, crushed
- Sixteen oz. fettuccine noodles, whole wheat
- One lb. mushrooms, sliced
- Four tbsp. margarine, separated
- One cup onion, chopped
- Two tbsp. whole wheat flour
- One and one-half lb. beef fillet steaks, lean
- Two tsp. Mustard, low-sodium
- One-half tsp. salt, separated
- Two cups vegetable broth, low-salt
- One tsp. paprika seasoning
- Three tsp. Worcestershire sauce, low-sodium
- One-half tsp. black pepper, separated
- Sixteen cups water
- One-third cup white wine, dry

Directions:

1. Prepare the onion by removing the skin and dicing it into small sections. Set aside.
2. Rub any extra dirt off of the mushrooms and slice. Set to the side.
3. Warm a deep pot with the water and the whole wheat fettuccine noodles with one-fourth teaspoon of the salt for approximately 10 minutes.
4. In the meantime, chop the beef into small cubes and dust with one-fourth teaspoon of pepper.
5. Liquefy two tablespoons of the margarine in a big skillet and transfer the cubed meat into the pan. Fry the meat for approximately 8 minutes while tossing occasionally to fully brown.
6. Remove the water from the cooked pasta and set to the side.
7. Use a spoon with holes to distribute the cooked meat to a platter and keep to the side.
8. Dissolve the leftover two tablespoons of margarine in the hot frying pan and fry the onions for approximately 5 minutes to caramelize.
9. Blend the garlic into the pan and heat for an additional half minute.
10. Then combine the mushrooms with the onions and fry for about 4 minutes.
11. Season the vegetables with the paprika and mustard and empty the wine into the skillet and heat for another 6 minutes, occasionally tossing and rubbing the base of the pan with a spatula that is wooden.

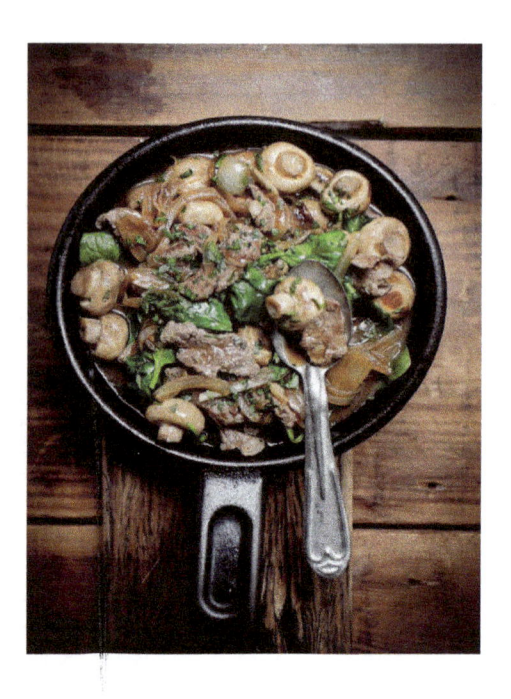

12. Meanwhile, blend the Worcestershire sauce, flour, and vegetable broth in a glass dish until there are no lumps present.
13. Empty the sauce into the skillet and bring to a slow bubble for approximately 5 minutes while occasionally stirring.
14. Transfer the cooked meat to the skillet and spice with the remaining one-fourth teaspoons of pepper and salt.
15. Turn the burner down to the setting of low and blend the sour cream into the skillet. Heat for an additional two minutes.
16. Distribute the cooked noodles into the pan and cover them fully with the sauce.
17. Spoon into serving dishes and enjoy immediately.

Nutrition:

- Sodium: 458 mg
- Protein: 42 g
- Fat: 11 g
- Sugar: 4 g
- Calories: 442

Pork Roast with Orange Sauce

Preparation Time: 15 minutes

Cooking Time: 80 minutes

Servings: 2

Ingredients:

- 1-pound pork loin roast
- ½ cup carrot, diced
- ½ cup celery stalk, chopped
- ½ cup onion, diced
- 1 teaspoon Italian seasonings
- 1 cup of orange juice
- 1 tablespoon potato starch

Directions:

1. Rub the pork loin roast with Italian seasonings.
2. Then put the carrot, celery stalk, and diced onion in the tray.
3. Put the meat over the vegetables. Add orange juice.
4. Bake the meat for 75 minutes at 365F.
5. After this, transfer all vegetables and juice to the saucepan and bring it to a boil.
6. Blend the mixture with the help of the blender. Add potato starch and whisk it well.
7. Simmer the sauce for 2 minutes.
8. Slice the cooked meat and sprinkle it with orange sauce.

Nutrition:

- 292 calories
- 33.2g protein
- 12.2g carbohydrates
- 11.4g fat
- 1g fiber
- 93mg cholesterol
- 87mg sodium

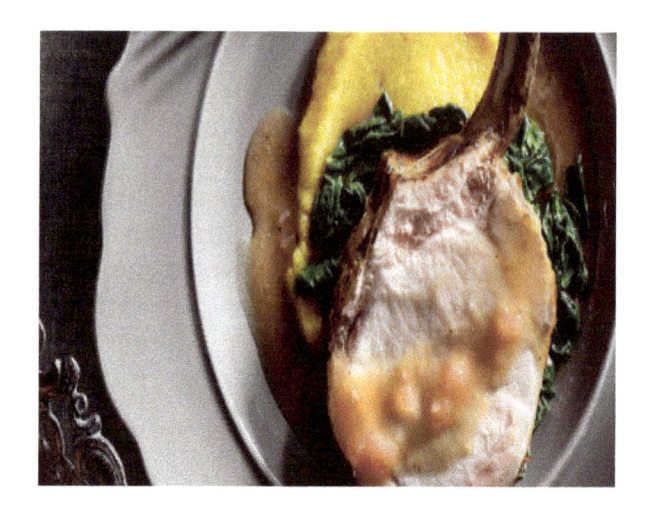

Southwestern Steak

Preparation Time: 15 minutes

Cooking Time: 16 minutes

Servings: 2

Ingredients:

- 2 beef flank steaks
- 1 tablespoon lemon juice
- 1 teaspoon chili flakes
- 1 teaspoon garlic powder
- 1 tablespoon avocado oil

Directions:

1. Preheat the grill to 385F.
2. Then rub the meat with chili flakes and garlic powder.
3. Then sprinkle it with lemon juice and avocado oil.
4. Grill the steaks for 8 minutes per side.

Nutrition:

- 174 calories
- 26.2g protein
- 1.6g carbohydrates
- 6.3g fat
- 0.5g fiber
- 76mg cholesterol
- 58mg sodium

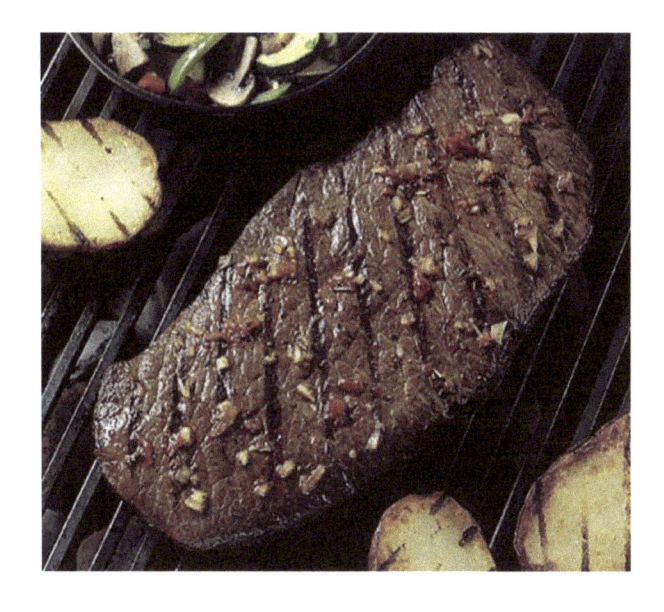

Tender Pork Medallions

Preparation Time: 10 minutes

Cooking Time: 25 minutes

Servings: 2

Ingredients:

- 12 oz pork tenderloin
- 1 teaspoon dried sage
- 1 tablespoon margarine
- 1 teaspoon ground black pepper
- ½ cup low-fat yogurt

Directions:

1. Cut the pork tenderloin into 3 medallions and sprinkle with sage and ground black pepper.
2. Heat up margarine in the saucepan and add pork medallions.
3. Roast them for 5 minutes per side.
4. Then add yogurt and coat the meat in it well.
5. Close the lid and simmer the medallions for 15 minutes over medium heat.

Nutrition:

- 227 calories
- 32.4g protein
- 3.5g carbohydrates
- 8.3g fat
- 0.3g fiber
- 85mg cholesterol
- 138mg sodium

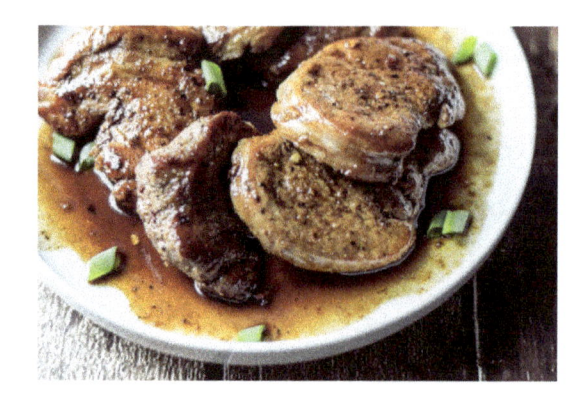

Garlic Pork Meatballs

Preparation Time: 10 minutes

Cooking Time: 28 minutes

Servings: 2

Ingredients:

- 2 pork medallions
- 1 teaspoon minced garlic
- ¼ cup of coconut milk
- 1 tablespoon olive oil
- 1 teaspoon cayenne pepper

Directions:

1. Sprinkle each pork medallion with cayenne pepper.
2. Heat up olive oil in the skillet and add meat.
3. Roast the pork medallions for 3 minutes from each side.
4. After this, add coconut milk and minced garlic. Close the lid and simmer the meat for 20 minutes on low heat.

Nutrition:

- 284 calories
- 25.9g protein
- 2.6g carbohydrates
- 18.8g fat
- 0.9g fiber
- 70mg cholesterol
- 60mg sodium

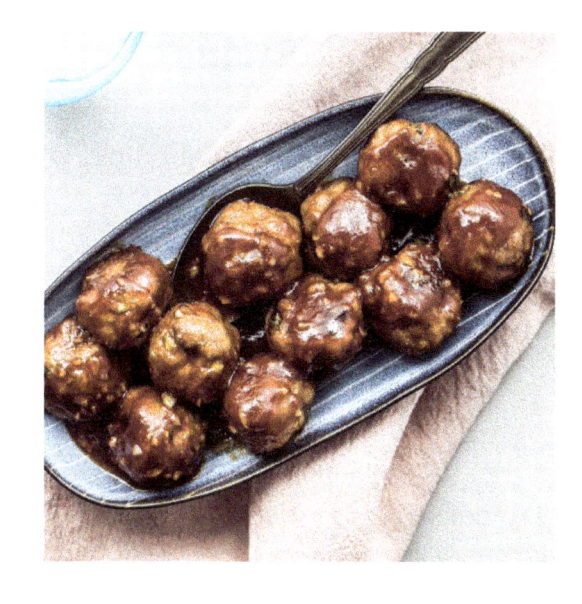

Fajita Pork Strips

Preparation Time: 10 minutes

Cooking Time: 35 minutes

Servings: 2

Ingredients:

- 16 oz pork sirloin
- 1 tablespoon Fajita seasonings
- 1 tablespoon canola oil

Directions:

1. Cut the pork sirloin into strips and sprinkle with fajita seasonings and canola oil.
2. Then transfer the meat to the baking tray in one layer.
3. Bake it for 35 minutes at 365F. Stir the meat every 10 minutes during cooking.

Nutrition:

- 184 calories
- 18.5g protein
- 1.3g carbohydrates
- 10.8g fat
- 0g fiber
- 64mg cholesterol
- 157mg sodium

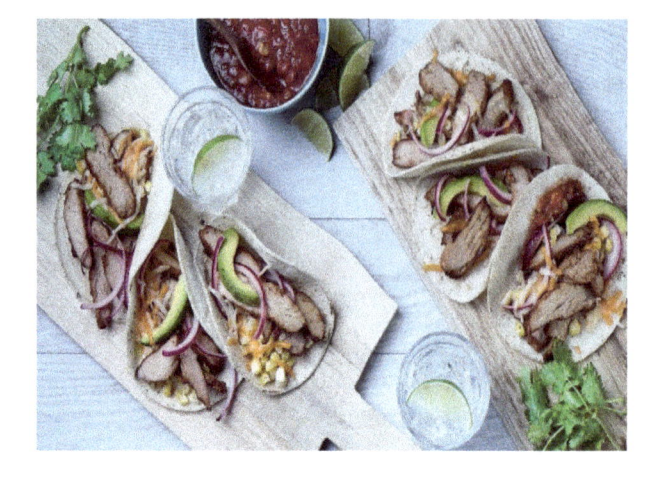

Pepper Pork Tenderloins

Preparation Time: 15 minutes

Cooking Time: 60 minutes

Servings: 2

Ingredients:

- 8 oz pork tenderloin
- 1 tablespoon mustard
- 1 teaspoon ground black pepper
- 2 tablespoons olive oil

Directions:

1. Rub the meat with mustard and sprinkle with ground black pepper.
2. Then brush it with olive oil and wrap it in the foil.
3. Bake the meat for 60 minutes at 375F.
4. Then discard the foil and slice the tenderloin into servings.

Nutrition:

- 311 calories
- 31.2g protein
- 2.6g carbohydrates
- 19.6g fat
- 1.1g fiber
- 83mg cholesterol
- 65mg sodium

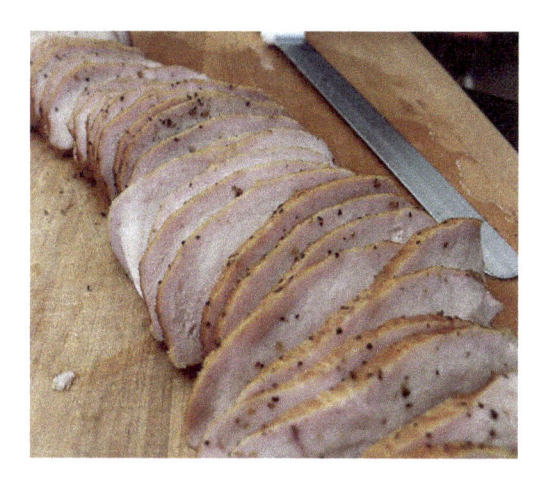

Spiced Beef

Preparation Time: 10 minutes

Cooking Time: 80 minutes

Servings: 2

Ingredients:

- 1-pound beef sirloin
- 1 tablespoon five-spice seasoning
- 1 bay leaf
- 2 cups of water
- 1 teaspoon peppercorn

Directions:

1. Rub the meat with five-spice seasoning and put it in the saucepan.
2. Add nay leaf, water, and peppercorns.
3. Close the lid and simmer it for 80 minutes on medium heat.
4. Chop the cooked meat and sprinkle it with hot spiced water from the saucepan.

Nutrition:

- 213 calories
- 34.5g protein
- 0.5g carbohydrates
- 7.1g fat
- 0.2g fiber
- 101mg cholesterol
- 116mg sodium

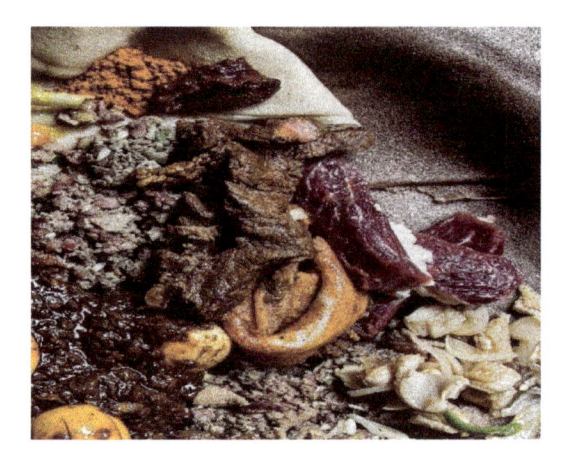

Tomato Beef

Preparation Time: 10 minutes

Cooking Time: 17 minutes

Servings: 2

Ingredients:

- 2 chuck shoulder steaks
- ¼ cup tomato sauce
- 1 tablespoon olive oil

Directions:

1. Brush the steaks with tomato sauce and olive oil and transfer to the preheated to 390F grill.
2. Grill the meat for 9 minutes.
3. Then flip it on another side and cook for 8 minutes more.

Nutrition:

- 247 calories
- 21.4g protein
- 1.7g carbohydrates
- 17.1g fat
- 0.5g fiber
- 70mg cholesterol
- 231mg sodium

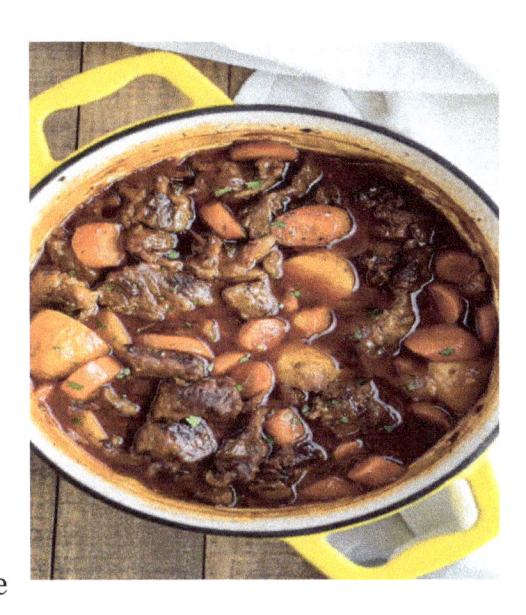

Hoisin Pork

Preparation Time: 10 minutes

Cooking Time: 14 minutes

Servings: 2

Ingredients:

- 1-pound pork loin steaks
- 2 tablespoons hoisin sauce
- 1 tablespoon apple cider vinegar
- 1 teaspoon olive oil

Directions:

1. Rub the pork steaks with hoisin sauce, apple cider vinegar, and olive oil.
2. Then preheat the grill to 395F.
3. Put the pork steak in the grill and cook them for 7 minutes per side.

Nutrition:

- 263 calories
- 39.3g protein
- 3.6g carbohydrates
- 10.1g fat
- 0.2g fiber
- 0mg cholesterol
- 130mg sodium

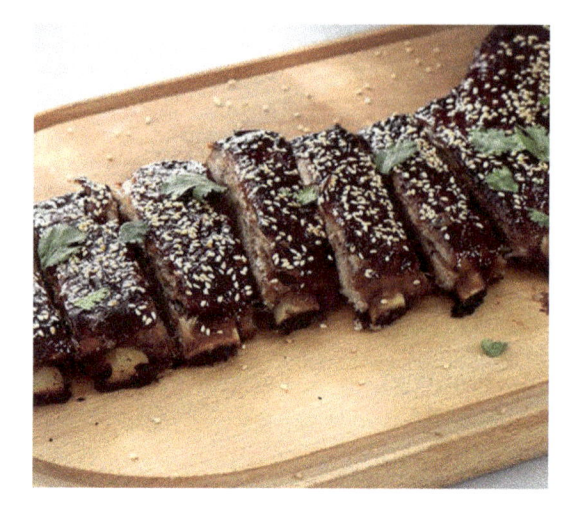

Sage Beef Loin

Preparation Time: 10 minutes

Cooking Time: 18 minutes

Servings: 2

Ingredients:

- 10 oz beef loin, strips
- 1 garlic clove, diced
- 2 tablespoons margarine
- 1 teaspoon dried sage

Directions:

1. Toss margarine in the skillet.
2. Add garlic and dried sage and roast them for 2 minutes on low heat.
3. Add beef loin strips and roast them for 15 minutes on medium heat. Stir the meat occasionally.

Nutrition:

- 363 calories
- 38.2g protein
- 0.8g carbohydrates
- 23.2g fat
- 0.2g fiber
- 101mg cholesterol
- 211mg sodium

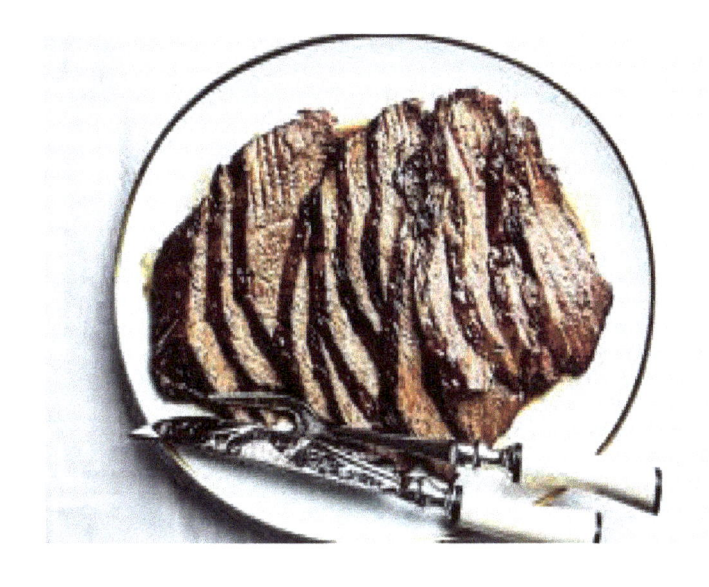

Beef Chili

Preparation Time: 10 minutes

Cooking Time: 30 minutes

Servings: 2

Ingredients:

- 1 cup lean ground beef
- 1 onion, diced
- 1 tablespoon olive oil
- 1 cup crushed tomatoes
- ½ cup red kidney beans, cooked
- ½ cup of water
- 1 teaspoon chili seasonings

Directions:

1. Heat up olive oil in the saucepan and add lean ground beef.
2. Cook it for 7 minutes over medium heat.
3. Then add chili seasonings and diced onion. Stir the ingredients and cook them for 10 minutes.
4. After this, add water, crushed tomatoes, red kidney beans, and stir the chili well.
5. Close the lid and simmer the meal for 13 minutes.

Nutrition:

- 220 calories
- 18.3g protein
- 22g carbohydrates
- 6.7g fat
- 6.1g fiber
- 34mg cholesterol
- 177mg sodium

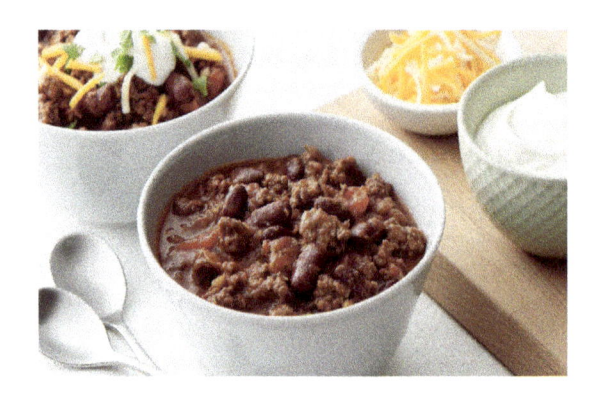

Celery Beef Stew

Preparation Time: 5 minutes

Cooking Time: 55 minutes

Servings: 2

Ingredients:

- 1-pound beef loin, chopped
- 2 cups celery stalk, chopped
- 1 garlic clove, diced
- 1 yellow onion, diced
- 1 tablespoon olive oil
- 1 tablespoon tomato paste
- 1 teaspoon chili powder
- 1 teaspoon dried dill
- 2 cups of water

Directions:

1. Roast the beef loin with olive oil in the saucepan for 5 minutes.
2. After this, add all remaining ingredients and close the lid.
3. Cook the stew for 50 minutes on medium heat.

Nutrition:

- 150 calories
- 14.6g protein
- 4.6g carbohydrates
- 7.9g fat
- 1.2g fiber
- 41mg cholesterol
- 370mg sodium

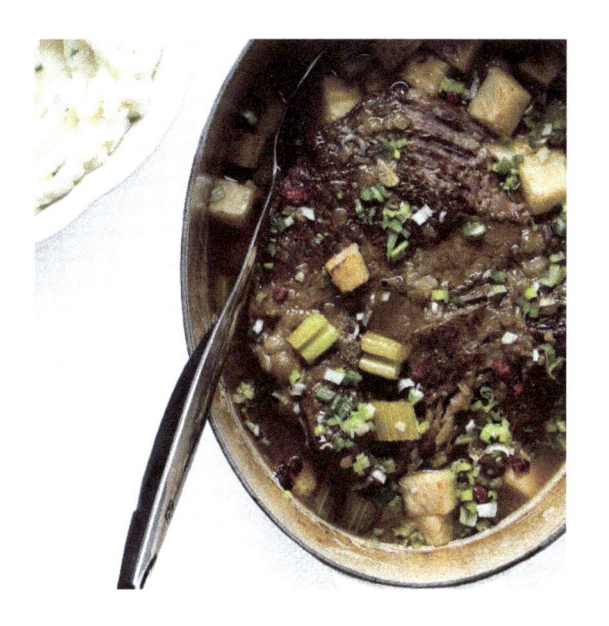

Beef Skillet

Preparation Time: 10 minutes

Cooking Time: 30 minutes

Servings: 2

Ingredients:

- 1 cup lean ground beef
- 1 cup bell pepper, sliced
- 2 tomatoes, chopped
- 1 chili pepper, chopped
- 1 tablespoon olive oil
- ½ cup of water

Directions:

1. Heat up olive oil in the skillet and add lean ground beef.
2. Roast it for 10 minutes.
3. Then stir the meat well and add chili pepper and bell pepper. Roast the ingredients for 10 minutes more.
4. Add tomatoes and water.
5. Close the lid and simmer the meal for 10 minutes.

Nutrition:

- 167 calories
- 16.1g protein
- 6.3g carbohydrates
- 8.8g fat
- 1.6g fiber
- 46mg cholesterol
- 50mg sodium

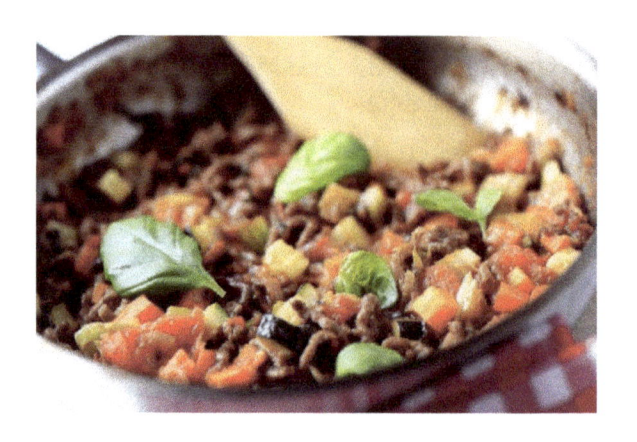

Hot Beef Strips

Preparation Time: 10 minutes

Cooking Time: 15 minutes

Servings: 2

Ingredients:

- 9 oz beef tenders
- 2 tablespoons cayenne pepper
- 1 tablespoon lemon juice
- 2 tablespoons canola oil

Directions:

1. Cut the beef tenders into strips and rub with cayenne pepper.
2. Sprinkle the meat with lemon juice and put it in the hot skillet.
3. Add canola oil and roast the meat for 15 minutes on medium heat. Stir it from time to time to avoid burning.

Nutrition:

- 231 calories
- 22.5g protein
- 2.1g carbohydrates
- 14.6g fat
- 1g fiber
- 54mg cholesterol
- 62mg sodium

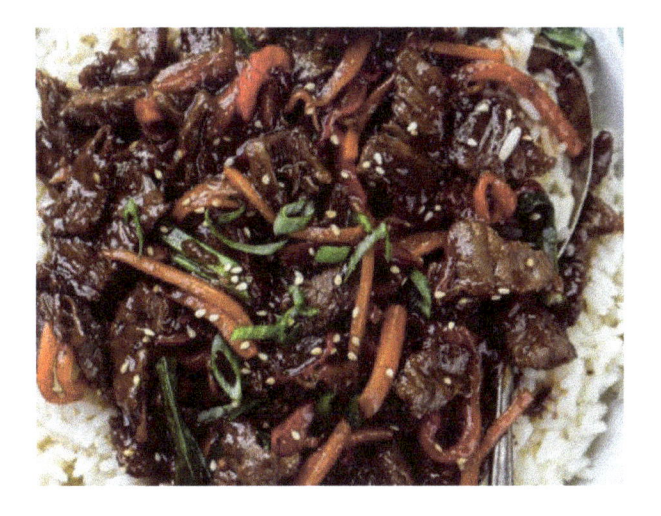

Sloppy Joe

Preparation Time: 10 minutes

Cooking Time: 35 minutes

Servings: 2

Ingredients:

- 1 cup lean ground beef
- 1 cup onion, diced
- ½ cup sweet peppers, diced
- 1 teaspoon minced garlic
- 1 tablespoon canola oil
- 1 teaspoon liquid honey
- ½ cup tomato puree
- 1 teaspoon tomato paste

Directions:

1. Mix up canola oil and lean ground beef in the saucepan.
2. Add onion and sweet pepper and stir the ingredient well.
3. Cook them for 10 minutes.
4. Then add honey, tomato puree, and tomato paste. Mix up the mixture well.
5. Close the lid and cook it for 25 minutes on medium heat.

Nutrition:

- 134 calories
- 7.6g protein
- 8.7g carbohydrates
- 7.7g fat
- 1.9g fiber
- 22mg cholesterol
- 34mg sodium

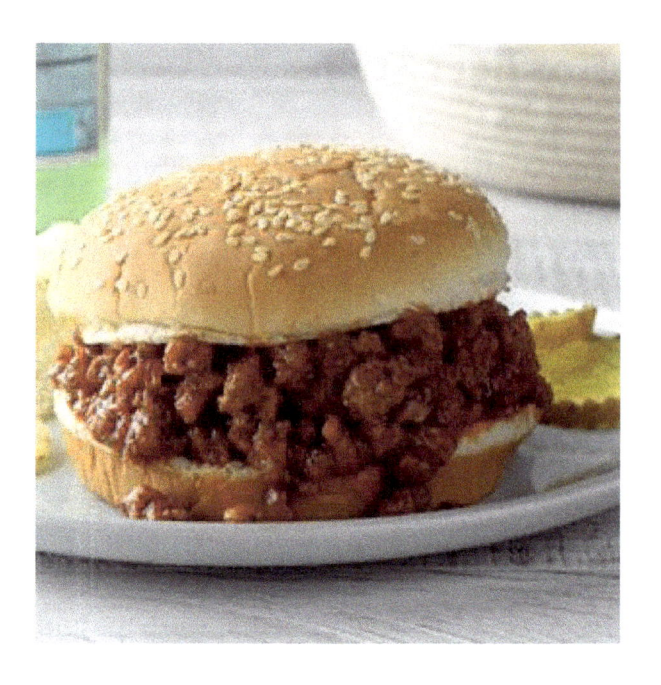

CHAPTER 8:

Snacks, Sides & Desserts

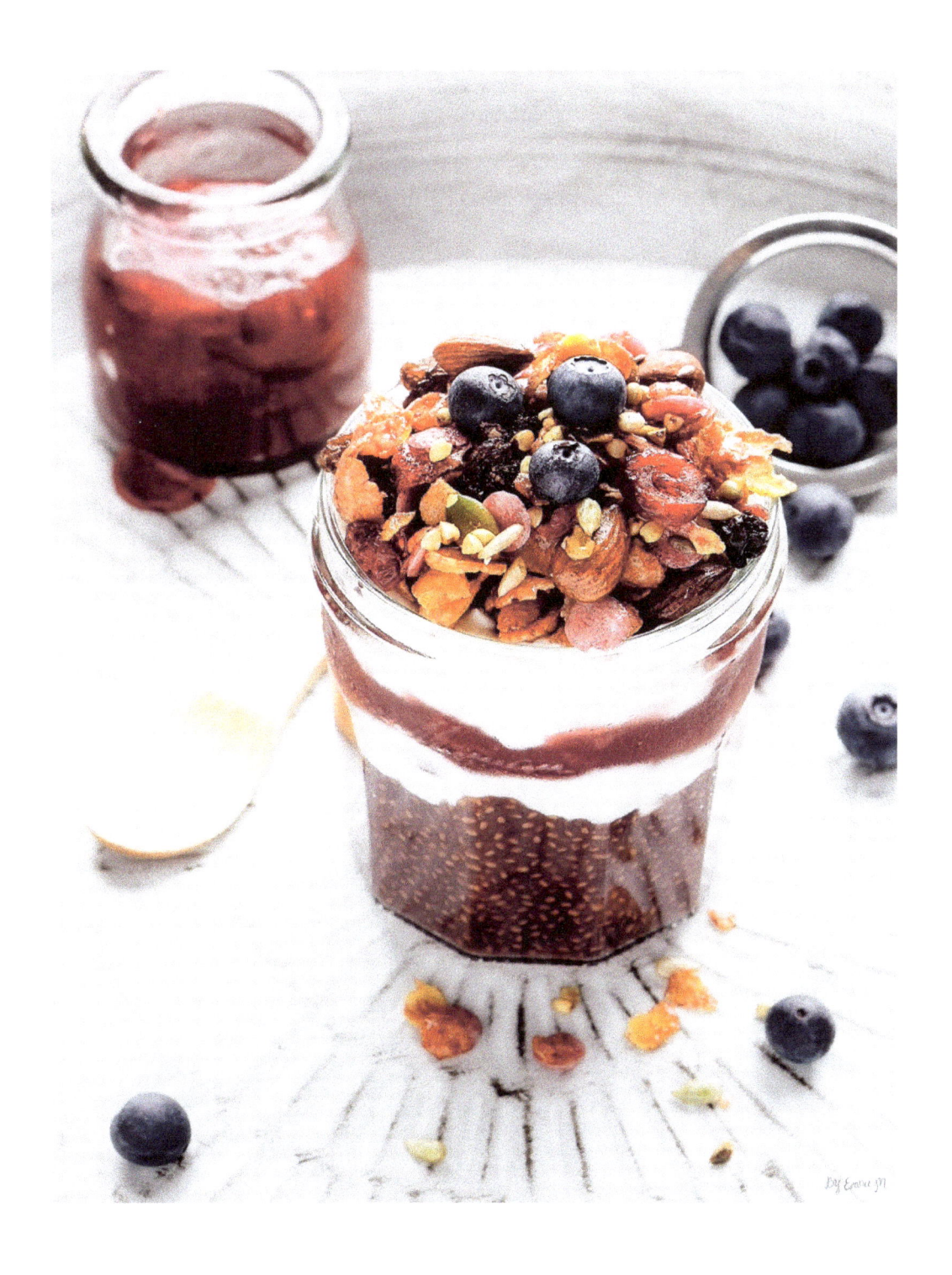

Summer Squash Ribbons with Lemon and Ricotta

Preparation Time: 20 minutes

Cooking Time: 0 minutes

Servings: 2

Ingredients:

- 2 medium zucchini or yellow squash
- ½ cup ricotta cheese
- 2 tablespoons fresh mint, chopped, plus additional mint leaves for garnish
- 2 tablespoons fresh parsley, chopped
- Zest of ½ lemon
- 2 teaspoons lemon juice
- ½ teaspoon kosher salt
- ¼ teaspoon freshly ground black pepper
- 1 tablespoon extra-virgin olive oil

Directions:

1. Using a vegetable peeler, make ribbons by peeling the summer squash lengthwise. The squash ribbons will resemble the wide pasta, pappardelle.
2. In a medium bowl, combine the ricotta cheese, mint, parsley, lemon zest, lemon juice, salt, and black pepper.
3. Place mounds of the squash ribbons evenly on 4 plates then dollop the ricotta mixture on top. Drizzle with olive oil and garnish with the mint leaves.

Nutrition:

- Calories: 90
- Total Fat: 6g
- Cholesterol: 10mg
- Sodium: 180mg
- Total Carbohydrates: 5g
- Fiber: 1g
- Sugars: 3g
- Protein: 5g

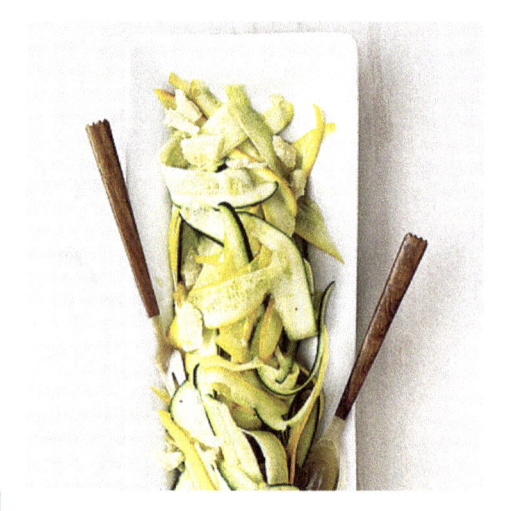

Sautéed Kale with Tomato and Garlic

Preparation Time: 5 minutes

Cooking Time: 10 minutes

Servings: 1

Ingredients:

- 1 tablespoon extra-virgin olive oil
- 4 garlic cloves, sliced
- ¼ teaspoon red pepper flakes
- 2 bunches kale, stemmed and chopped or torn into pieces
- 1 (14.5-ounce) can no-salt-added diced tomatoes
- ½ teaspoon kosher salt

Directions:

1. Heat the olive oil in a wok or large skillet over medium-high heat. Add the garlic and red pepper flakes, and sauté until fragrant, about 30 seconds. Add the kale and sauté, about 3 to 5 minutes, until the kale shrinks down a bit.
2. Add the tomatoes and the salt, stir together, and cook for 3 to 5 minutes, or until the liquid reduces and the kale cooks down further and becomes tender.

Nutrition:

- Calories: 110
- Total Fat: 5g
- Cholesterol: 0mg
- Sodium: 222mg
- Total Carbohydrates: 15g
- Fiber: 6g
- Sugars: 6g
- Protein: 6g

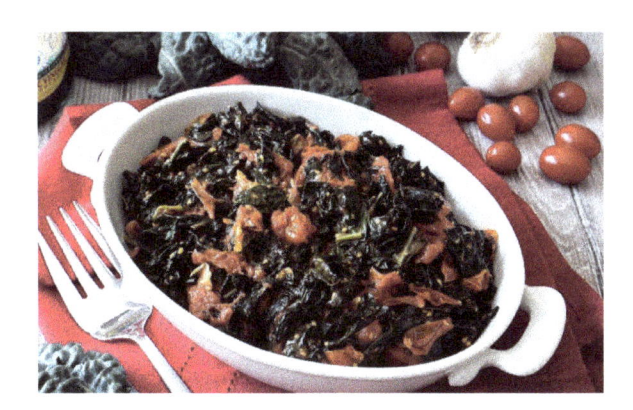

Roasted Broccoli with Tahini Yogurt Sauce

Preparation Time: 15 minutes

Cooking Time: 30 minutes

Servings: 2

Ingredients:

- 1½ to 2 pounds broccoli, stalk trimmed and cut into slices, head cut into florets
- 1 lemon, sliced into ¼-inch-thick rounds
- 3 tablespoons extra-virgin olive oil
- ½ teaspoon kosher salt
- ¼ teaspoon freshly ground black pepper
- ½ cup plain Greek yogurt
- 2 tablespoons tahini
- 1 tablespoon lemon juice
- ¼ teaspoon kosher salt
- 1 teaspoon sesame seeds, for garnish (optional)

Directions:

1. Preheat the oven to 425°F. Line a baking sheet with parchment paper or foil.
2. In a large bowl, gently toss the broccoli, lemon slices, olive oil, salt, and black pepper to combine. Arrange the broccoli in a single layer on the prepared baking sheet. Roast 15 minutes, stir, and roast another 15 minutes, until golden brown.

To Make The Tahini Yogurt Sauce:

1. In a medium bowl, combine the yogurt, tahini, lemon juice, and salt; mix well.
2. Spread the tahini yogurt sauce on a platter or large plate and top with the broccoli and lemon slices. Garnish with the sesame seeds (if desired).

Nutrition:

- Calories: 245
- Total Fat: 16g
- Cholesterol: 2mg
- Sodium: 305mg
- Total Carbohydrates: 20g
- Fiber: 7g
- Sugars: 6g
- Protein: 12g

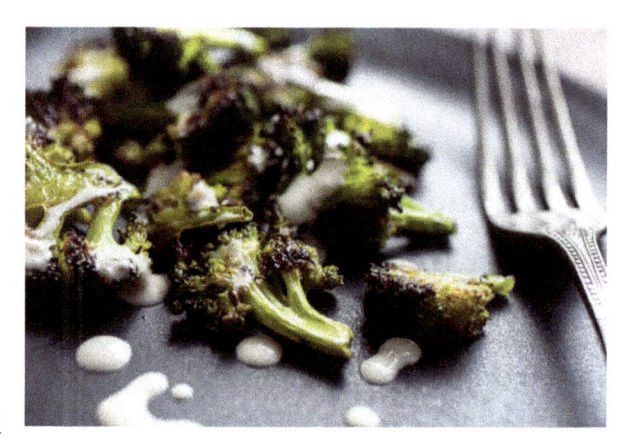

Green Beans with Pine Nuts and Garlic

Preparation Time: 10 minutes

Cooking Time: 20 minutes

Servings: 1-2

Ingredients:

- 1 pound green beans, trimmed
- 1 head garlic (10 to 12 cloves), smashed
- 2 tablespoons extra-virgin olive oil
- ½ teaspoon kosher salt
- ¼ teaspoon red pepper flakes
- 1 tablespoon white wine vinegar
- ¼ cup pine nuts, toasted

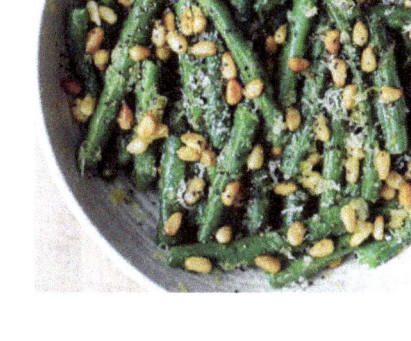

Directions:

1. Preheat the oven to 425°F. Line a baking sheet with parchment paper or foil.
2. In a large bowl, combine the green beans, garlic, olive oil, salt, and red pepper flakes and mix. Arrange in a single layer on the baking sheet. Roast for 10 minutes, stir, and roast for another 10 minutes, or until golden brown.
3. Mix the cooked green beans with the vinegar and top with the pine nuts.

Nutrition:

- Calories: 165
- Total Fat: 13g
- Cholesterol: 0mg
- Sodium: 150mg
- Total Carbohydrates: 12g
- Fiber: 4g
- Sugars: 4g
- Protein: 4g

Roasted Harissa Carrots

Preparation Time: 10 minutes

Cooking Time: 15 minutes

Servings: 2

Ingredients:

- 1 pound carrots, peeled and sliced into 1-inch-thick rounds
- 2 tablespoons extra-virgin olive oil
- 2 tablespoons harissa
- 1 teaspoon honey
- 1 teaspoon ground cumin
- ½ teaspoon kosher salt
- ½ cup fresh parsley, chopped

Directions:

1. Preheat the oven to 450°F. Line a baking sheet with parchment paper or foil.
2. In a large bowl, combine the carrots, olive oil, harissa, honey, cumin, and salt. Arrange in a single layer on the baking sheet. Roast for 15 minutes. Remove from the oven, add the parsley, and toss together.

Nutrition:

- Calories: 120
- Total Fat: 8g
- Cholesterol: 0mg
- Sodium: 255mg
- Total Carbohydrates: 13g
- Fiber: 4g
- Sugars: 7g
- Protein: 1g

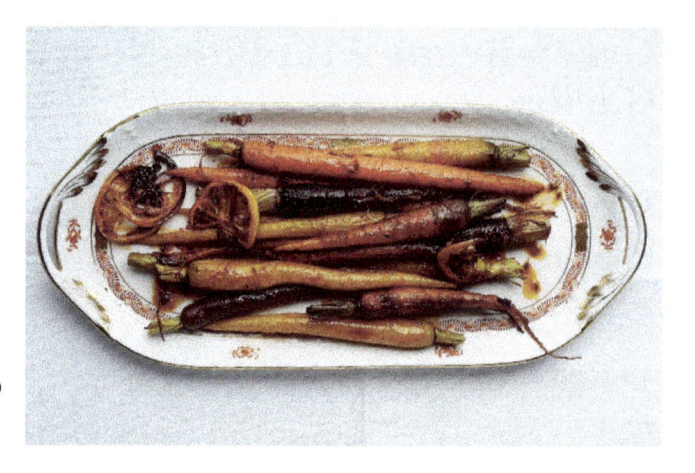

Toasted Almond Ambrosia

Preparation Time: 30 minutes

Cooking Time: 0 minutes

Servings: 2

Ingredients:

- ½ cup almonds, slivered
- ½ cup coconut, shredded & unsweetened
- 3 cups pineapple, cubed
- 5 oranges, cut
- 1 banana, halved lengthwise, peeled & sliced
- 2 red apples, cored & diced
- 2 tablespoons cream sherry
- mint leaves, fresh to garnish

Directions:

1. Start by heating your oven to 325, and then get out a baking sheet. Roast your almonds for ten minutes, making sure they're spread out evenly.
2. Transfer them to a plate and then toast your coconut on the same baking sheet. Toast for ten minutes.
3. Mix your banana, sherry, oranges, apples, and pineapple in a bowl.
4. Divide the mixture not serving bowls and top with coconut and almonds.
5. Garnish with mint before serving.

Nutrition:

- Calories: 177
- Protein: 3.4 g
- Fat: 4.9 g
- Carbs: 36 g
- Sodium: 13 mg
- Cholesterol: 11 mg

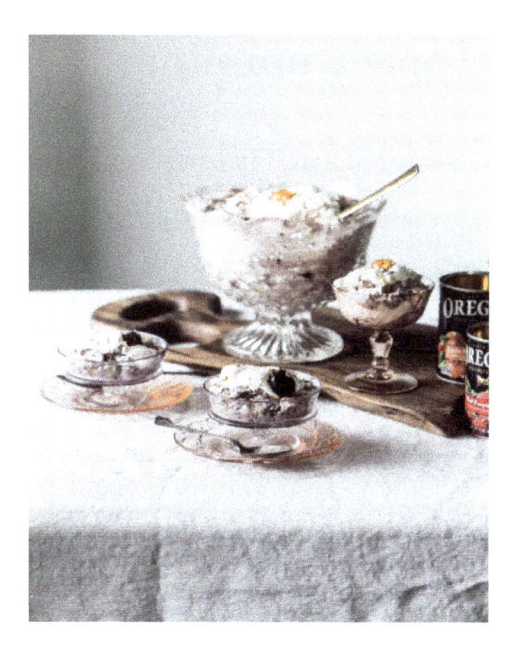

Apple Dumplings

Preparation Time: 40 minutes

Cooking Time: 0 minutes

Servings: 2

Ingredients:

Dough:

- 1 tablespoon butter
- 1 teaspoon honey, raw
- 1 cup whole wheat flour
- 2 tablespoons buckwheat flour
- 2 tablespoons rolled oats
- 2 tablespoons brandy or apple liquor

Filling:

- 2 tablespoons honey, raw
- 1 teaspoon nutmeg
- 6 tart apples, sliced thin
- 1 lemon, zested

Directions:

1. Turn the oven to 350. Get out a food processor and mix your butter, flours, honey, and oats until it forms a crumbly mixture. Add in your brandy or apple liquor, pulsing until it forms a dough.
2. Seal in plastic and place it in the fridge for two hours.
3. Toss your apples in lemon zest, honey, and nutmeg.
4. Roll your dough into a sheet that's a quarter-inch thick. Cut out eight-inch circles, placing each circle into a muffin tray that's been greased.
5. Press the dough down and then stuff with the apple mixture. Fold the edges, and pinch them closed. Make sure that they're well sealed.
6. Bake for a half-hour until golden brown, and serve drizzled in honey.

Nutrition:

- Calories: 178
- Protein: 5 g
- Fat: 4 g
- Carbs: 23 g
- Sodium: 562 mg
- Cholesterol: 61 mg

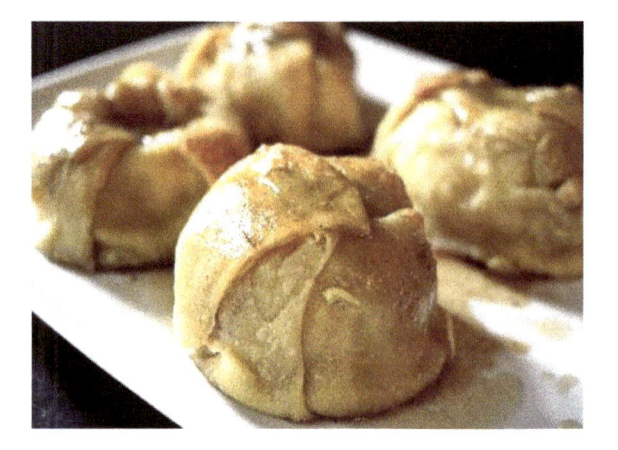

Almond Rice Pudding

Preparation Time: 25 minutes

Cooking Time: 20 minutes

Servings: 2

Ingredients:

- 3 cups 1% milk
- 1 cup white rice
- ¼ cup sugar
- 1 teaspoon vanilla
- ¼ teaspoon almond extract
- Cinnamon
- ¼ cup toasted almonds

Directions:

1. Combine milk and rice in a medium saucepan. Bring them to a boil.
2. Reduce heat and simmer for 20 minutes with the lid on until the rice is soft.
3. Remove from heat and add the sugar, vanilla, almond extract, and cinnamon.
4. Sprinkle toasted almonds on top and serve warm.

Nutrition:

- Calories 180
- Total fat 1.5 g
- Carbohydrates 36 g
- Protein 7 g
- Fiber 1 g
- Sodium 65 mg

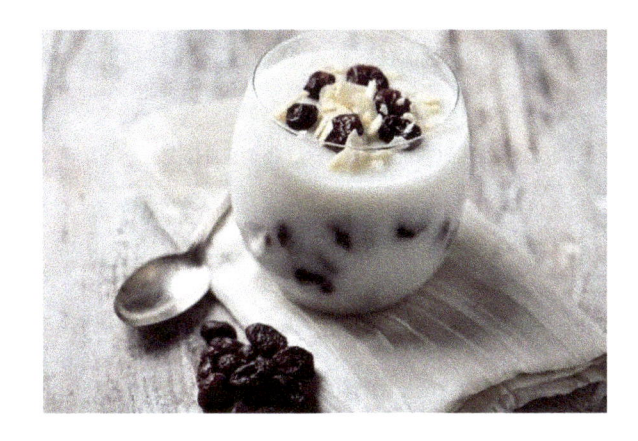

Apples and Cream Shake

Preparation Time: 10 minutes

Cooking Time: 0 minutes

Servings: 1

Ingredients:

- 2 cups vanilla low fat ice cream
- 1 cup apple sauce
- 1/4 teaspoon ground cinnamon
- 1 cup fat-free skim milk

Directions:

1. In a blender container combine the low-fat ice cream, applesauce, and cinnamon. Cover and blend until smooth.
2. Add fat-free skim milk. Cover and blend until mixed.
3. Pour into glasses.
4. Serve immediately.

Nutrition:

- Calories 160
- Total fat 3 g
- Carbohydrates 27 g
- Protein 6 g
- Fiber 1 g
- Sodium 80 mg

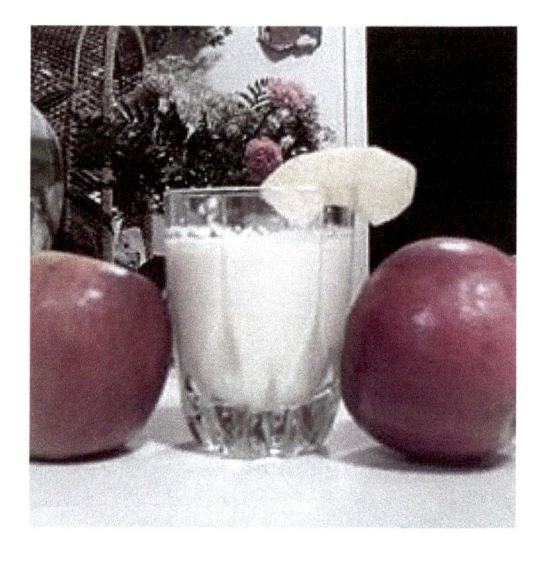

Baked Stuffed Apples

Preparation Time: 10 minutes

Cooking Time: 8 minutes

Servings: 2

Ingredients:

- 4 Jonagold apples
- 1/4 cup flaked coconut
- 1/4 cup chopped dried apricots
- 2 teaspoons grated orange zest
- 1/2 cup orange juice
- 2 tablespoons brown sugar

Directions:

1. Peel top 1/3 of apples and hollow out center with a knife. Arrange, peeled end up, in a microwave-safe baking dish. Combine coconut, apricots, and orange zest. Divide to evenly fill centers of apples.
2. Mix orange juice and brown sugar. Pour over apples. Cover tightly with vented plastic wrap and microwave on high for 8 minutes or until apples are tender. Cool before serving.

Nutrition:

- Calories 192
- Total fat 2 g
- Carbohydrates 46 g
- Protein 1 g
- Fiber 6 g
- Sodium 19 mg

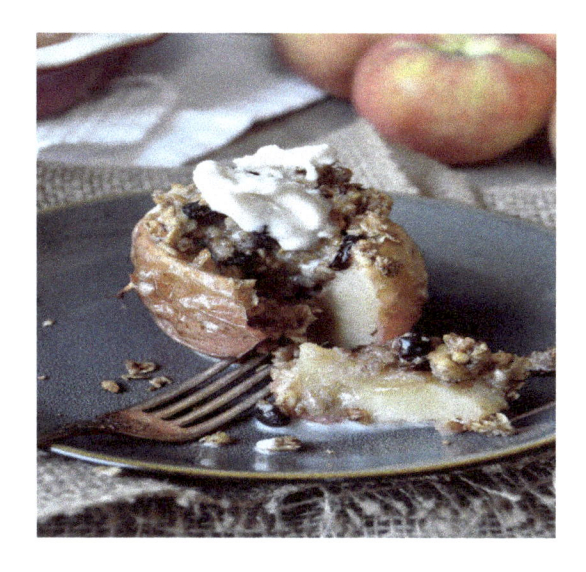

Apricot Biscotti

Preparation Time: 50 minutes

Cooking Time: 0 minutes

Servings: 2

Ingredients:

- 2 tablespoons honey, dark
- 2 tablespoons olive oil
- ½ teaspoon almond extract
- ¼ cup almonds, chopped roughly
- 2/3 cup apricots, dried
- 2 tablespoons milk, 1% & low fat
- 2 eggs, beaten lightly
- ¾ cup whole wheat flour
- ¾ cup all-purpose flour
- ¼ cup brown sugar, packed firm
- 1 teaspoon baking powder

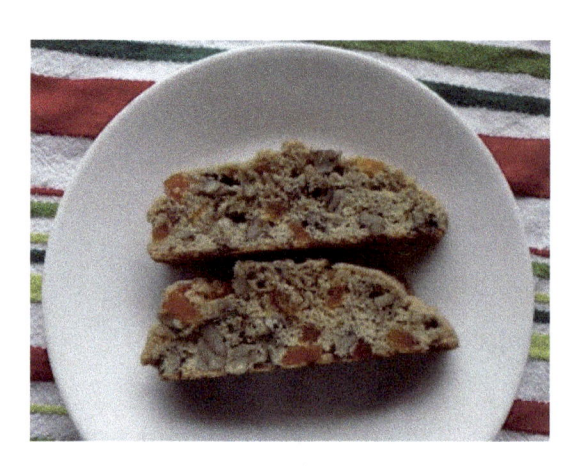

Directions:

1. Start by heating the oven to 350, and then mix your baking powder, brown sugar, and flours in a bowl.
2. Whisk your canola oil, eggs, almond extract, honey, and milk. Mix well until it forms a smooth dough. Fold in the apricots and almonds.
3. Put your dough on plastic wrap, and then roll it out to a twelve-inch long and three-inch wide rectangle. Place this dough on a baking sheet, and bake for twenty-five minutes. It should turn golden brown. Allow it to cool, and slice it into ½ inch thick slices, and then bake for another fifteen minutes. It should be crispy.

Nutrition:

- Calories: 291
- Protein: 2 g
- Fat: 2 g
- Carbs: 12 g
- Sodium: 123 mg
- Cholesterol: 21 mg

Apple & Berry Cobbler

Preparation Time: 40 minutes

Cooking Time: 0 minutes

Servings: 2

Ingredients:

Filling:

- 1 cup blueberries, fresh
- 2 cups apples, chopped
- 1 cup raspberries, fresh
- 2 tablespoons brown sugar
- 1 teaspoon lemon zest
- 2 teaspoon lemon juice, fresh
- ½ teaspoon ground cinnamon
- 1 ½ tablespoons corn starch

Topping:

- ¾ cup whole wheat pastry flour
- 1 ½ tablespoons brown sugar
- ½ teaspoon vanilla extract, pure
- ¼ cup soy milk
- ¼ teaspoon sea salt, fine
- 1 egg white

Directions:

1. Turn your oven to 350, and get out six small ramekins. Grease them with cooking spray. Mix your lemon juice, lemon zest, blueberries, sugar, cinnamon, raspberries, and apples together in a bowl.
2. Stir in your cornstarch, mixing until it dissolves.
3. Beat your egg white in a different bowl, whisking it with sugar, vanilla, soy milk, and pastry flour.
4. Divide your berry mixture between the ramekins and top with the vanilla topping.
5. Put your ramekins on a baking sheet, baking for thirty minutes. The top should be golden brown before serving.

Nutrition:

- Calories: 131 Protein: 7.2 g
- Fat: 1 g Carbs: 13.8 g Sodium: 14 mg Cholesterol: 2.1 mg

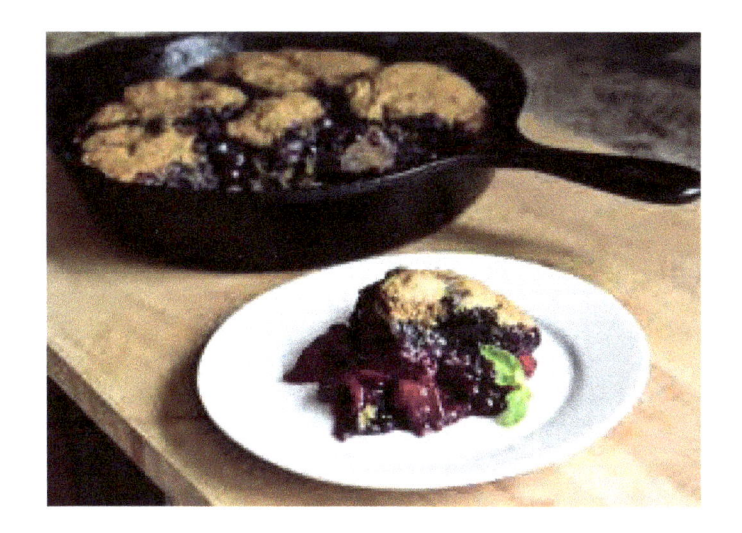

Mixed Fruit Compote Cups

Preparation Time: 15minutes

Cooking Time: 0 minutes

Servings: 2

Ingredients:

- 1 ¼ cup water
- ½ cup orange juice
- 12 ounces mixed dried fruit
- 1 teaspoon ground cinnamon
- ¼ teaspoon ground ginger
- ¼ teaspoon ground nutmeg
- 4 cups vanilla frozen yogurt, fat-free

Directions:

1. Mix your dried fruit, nutmeg, cinnamon, water, orange juice, and ginger in a saucepan.
2. Cover, and allow it to cook over medium heat for ten minutes. Remove the cover, and then cook for another ten minutes.
3. Add your frozen yogurt to serving cups, and top with the fruit mixture.

Nutrition:

- Calories: 228
- Protein: 9.1 g
- Fat: 5.7 g
- Carbs: 12.4 g
- Sodium: 114 mg
- Cholesterol: 15 mg

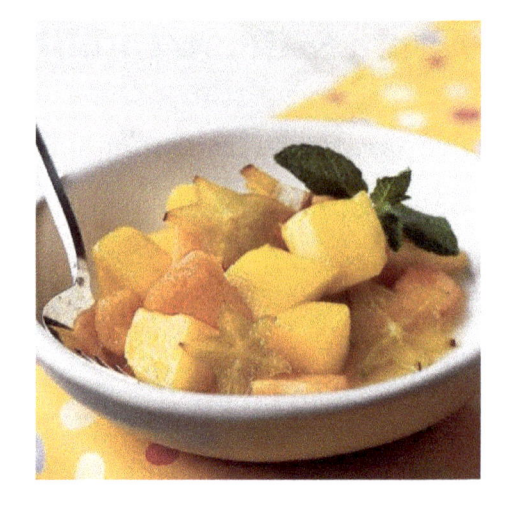

Oatmeal Surprise Cookies

Preparation Time: 25 minutes

Cooking Time: 0 minutes

Servings: 2

Ingredients:

- 1 ½ cups creamy peanut butter, all natural
- ½ cup dark brown sugar
- 2 eggs, large
- 1 cup old fashioned rolled oats
- 1 teaspoon baking soda
- ½ teaspoon sea salt, fine
- ½ cup dark chocolate chips

Directions:

1. Start by heating your oven to 350, and get out a baking sheet. Line your baking sheet with parchment paper.
2. Get out a bowl with an electric mixer and whip your peanut butter until smooth. Continue beating as you add in your brown sugar. Keep beating as you add in one egg at a time until it's incorporated and fluffy. Beat in your oats, salt, and baking soda. Turn the mixer off and fold in your dark chocolate chips.
3. Put your cookie dough on a baking sheet two inches apart and bake for eight to ten minutes.

Nutrition:

- Calories: 152
- Protein: 4 g
- Fat: 10 g
- Carbs: 12 g
- Sodium: 131 mg
- Cholesterol: 18 mg

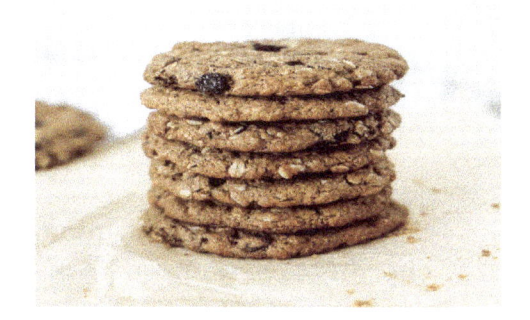

Almond & Apricot Crisp

Preparation Time: 35 minutes

Cooking Time: 0 minutes

Servings: 2

Ingredients:

- 1 teaspoon olive oil
- 1 lb. Apricot, halved & pits removed
- ½ cup almonds, chopped
- 1 tablespoons oats
- 1 teaspoon anise seeds
- 2 tablespoons honey, raw

Directions:

1. Start by heating the oven to 350, and then grease a nine-inch pie plate with olive oil.
2. Add in your apricots once they're chopped, and spread them out evenly.
3. Top with anise seeds, oats, and almonds. Pour honey on top, and bake for twenty-five minutes. It should turn golden brown.

Nutrition:

- Calories: 149
- Protein: 3 g
- Fat: 11.9 g
- Carbs: 18.8 g
- Sodium: 79 mg
- Cholesterol: 78 mg

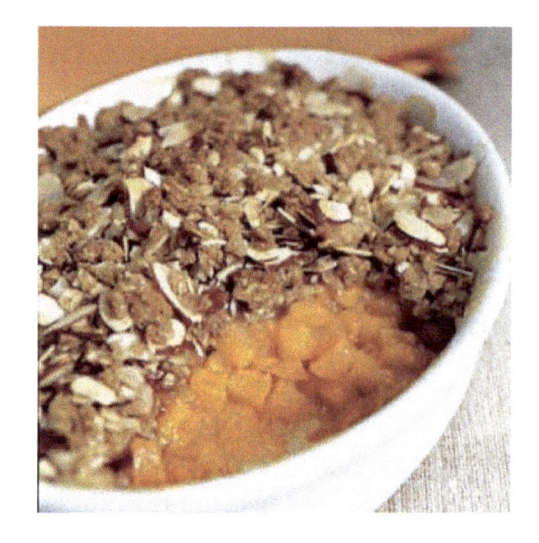

Blueberry Apple Cobbler

Preparation Time: 40 minutes

Cooking Time: 0 minutes

Servings: 2

Ingredients:

- 2 tablespoons cornstarch
- 2 tablespoons sugar
- 1 tablespoon lemon juice, fresh
- 2 apples, large, peeled, cored & sliced
- 1 teaspoon ground cinnamon
- 12 ounces blueberries, fresh

Toppings:

- ¼ teaspoon sea salt, fine
- ¾ cup all-purpose flour
- ¾ cup whole wheat flour
- 2 tablespoons sugar
- 1 ½ teaspoons baking powder
- 4 tablespoons margarine, cold & chopped
- ½ cup milk, fat-free
- 1 teaspoon vanilla extract, pure

Directions:

1. Turn the oven to 400 degrees, and then get out a nine-inch baking pan. Grease it using cooking spray. Mix your lemon juice and apples in a bowl before adding in your cornstarch, sugar, and cinnamon. Make sure it's evenly coated.
2. Toss the blueberries in, and then spread the mixture into the baking dish.
3. Get out a bowl and mix baking powder, both flours, sugar, and salt together.
4. Cut the margarine and mix it in until it forms a crumbly dough.
5. Stir in the milk and vanilla, and mix well to form a moist dough.
6. Knead with floured hands. Roll it out into a half an inch-thick rectangle.
7. Cut the dough into your favorite shapes using a cookie cutter.
8. Use the remaining scraps to cut more cookies.
9. Place this on top of your apple mixture until it is completely covered, and bake for a half-hour before serving.

Nutrition:

- Calories: 288 Protein: 6 g Fat: 6.2 g Carbs: 48 g Sodium: 176 mg
- Cholesterol: 120 mg

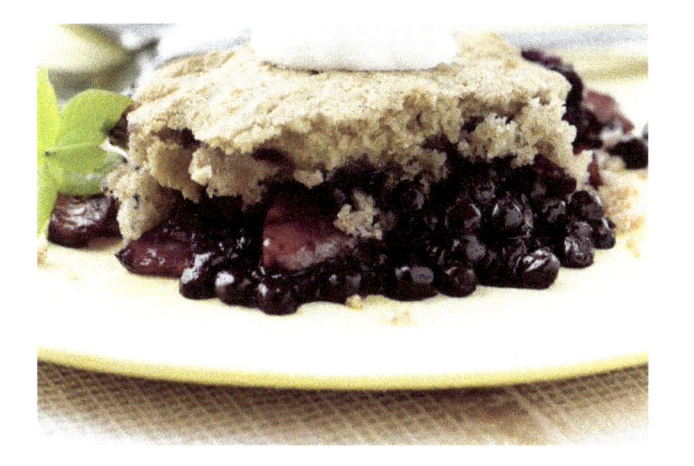

CHAPTER 9:

Measurement Conversions

Measurement

Cup	Ounces	Milliliters	Tablespoons
8 cups	64 oz	1895 ml	128
6 cups	48 oz	1420 ml	96
5 cups	40 oz	1180 ml	80
4 cups	32 oz	960 ml	64
2 cups	16 oz	480 ml	32
1 cup	8 oz	240 ml	16
3/4 cup	6 oz	177 ml	12
2/3 cup	5 oz	158 ml	11
1/2 cup	4 oz	118 ml	8
3/8 cup	3 oz	90 ml	6
1/3 cup	2.5 oz	79 ml	5.5
1/4 cup	2 oz	59 ml	4
1/8 cup	1 oz	30 ml	3
1/16 cup	1/2 oz	15 ml	1

Weight

Imperial	Metric
1/2 oz	15 g
1 oz	29 g
2 oz	57 g
3 oz	85 g
4 oz	113 g
5 oz	141 g
6 oz	170 g
8 oz	227 g
10 oz	283 g
12 oz	340 g
13 oz	369 g
14 oz	397 g
15 oz	425 g
1 lb	453 g

Temperature

Fahrenheit	Celsius
100 °F	37 °C
150 °F	65 °C
200 °F	93 °C
250 °F	121 °C
300 °F	150 °C
325 °F	160 °C
350 °F	180 °C
375 °F	190 °C
400 °F	200 °C
425 °F	220 °C
450 °F	230 °C
500 °F	260 °C
525 °F	274 °C
550 °F	288 °C

Conclusion

Statistics have it that one in three people have hypertension in America, and those that have normal blood pressure at the age of 50 or so have a 90% chance of getting affected in the near future. This is a high number considering how dangerous to your health hypertension can be. Having hypertension also means that you are prone to other health-related illnesses and diseases and this means an unhealthy life, and sometimes a short life.

This is not something that you cannot avoid though because making the right dietary choices has been seen to work really well to improve the health of people as well as reduce chances of suffering from hypertension and other health-related issues. The right choices can also make the existing condition manageable and you can still enjoy a longer, healthier life thereafter.

It is not too late to venture into a DASH Diet, a diet plan that will bring major changes in your health and life in general. This, along with staying active, limiting alcohol consumption, controlling your body weight, and staying stress-free will help a lot in enjoying a long happy life.

DASH diet is very easy to follow as it is the easiest diet plan so far but if you have to make huge diet changes. In order to fully adapt the DASH diet in your life, it is good to start making small changes bit by bit. Replace some of the unhealthy foods with healthy foods one day at a time. It will not be hard to stick to the diet plan this way. Convince your mind that healthy foods are the right foods to eat at all times and always have these healthy foods at your disposal in the place of unhealthy ones.

Lightning Source UK Ltd.
Milton Keynes UK
UKHW050815190221
378928UK00004B/24